APPRECIATION F

HEART TO SOUL CARDI~~~~ ~~~~~~~~

"There is so much credible wisdom in *Heart to Soul Cardiac Wellness*! Mary's insight as a cardiac ICU nurse, and her commitment to prevention from a truly holistic approach is a gift for anyone who wants to protect their own and their family's well-being. You'll find lots of things to learn, great tips to use, and resources to help guide you through a practical, personal plan to protect your heart, and overall health, which so many people don't really know how to do."

—DR. ILANA ZABLOZKI-AMIR,
Brooklyn Integrative Medicine, Brooklyn, NY

"*Heart to Soul Cardiac Wellness* is a must have resource for cardiac patients and their families. It is full of actionable items and interactive guides. The case-based discussions make cardiac disease and its risk factors understandable and relatable. We are long overdue for a resource like this!"

—HAFIZA H. KHAN, MD, FACC, FHRS, Clinical Cardiac
Electrophysiologist, Baylor Scott and White Health, Plano, Texas

"If you prefer *not to be* one of the nearly 650,000 Americans who die from heart disease annually, that's 1 in every 4 deaths, then *Heart to Soul Cardiac Wellness* is your path to personal empowerment. This unique book puts Mary Yuter—an experienced cardiac nurse certified in critical care, whole food plant-based nutrition, and cardiac medical yoga—at your side with clear, practical, and easy to implement advice to foster health and wellness. You'll learn about the "Cardiac Bermuda Triangle" (high blood pressure, high cholesterol and fats, and high blood sugar), Living your Life on the Veg with food as medicine, and how to prepare and recover from cardiac surgery, if relevant. As a lifestyle medicine proponent and one of Castle Connolly's America's Top Doctors for over 20 years, I enthusiastically endorse this inspiring and evidence-based guide to personal longevity."

–RICHARD M. ROSENFELD, MD, MPH, MBA,
Distinguished Professor and Chairman of Otolaryngology,
Founder and Chair, Committee on Plant-based Health and Nutrition,
SUNY Downstate Health Sciences University, Brooklyn, NY, USA

"Unlike others who attempt to educate readers on the importance of cardiovascular health, Mary is able to comprehensively incorporate the expectations and management of cardiovascular disease with the importance of self-motivation and awareness. It is truly a manual of health, identifying a holistic strategy of mental and physical health. It leaves readers empowered for managing their health with a unique stepwise approach through a two-month journey to revolutionize your wellness. As a practicing cardiologist who values the role of diet and lifestyle in disease prevention, I highly recommend this book to anyone at risk or actively dealing with cardiovascular needs."

–HEATH WILT, DO, FACC, Co-Founder ABCs of Health Cardiologist,
Noninvasive Imaging Director and Cardiac Rehab Director,
Advent Health-Shawnee Mission Medical Center, Merriam, KS

"This book is so inspiring! Once I picked up *Heart to Soul Cardiac Wellness*, I genuinely could not put it down because I felt like I was learning something new on every single page. *Heart to Soul Cardiac Wellness* doesn't feel like an onerous commitment to the reader as cardiac health, like any lifestyle change, usually seems to be. The information shared is given at the reader's pace and spread out over time to allow people to focus on making one change at a time and committing to that change through the covenant provided. In my opinion, this guide goes above and beyond cardiac health and really touches on some key indispensable aspects of health and wellness that the modern world has totally forgotten about."

—S. C., New York, New York

"*Heart to Soul Cardiac Wellness* is very relatable, encouraging, and easy to understand. It will empower you to listen to your body, and support and encourage you as you learn tips about how to do your best to prevent heart disease. Mary guides you to start each day with breath work and mediation and end your day with gratitude reflection. This book should be in the hands of every patient who wants to have a positive attitude while overcoming heart conditions. I confidently recommend *Heart to Soul Cardiac Wellness*. Get ready to shift your mindset to positivity and take control of YOU!"

—NICOLE WILT, LLC ABC's of Health, B.S. Kinesiology,
    Certified Personal Trainer & Yoga Instructor, Prairie Village, KS

"What's so indispensable about *Heart to Soul Cardiac Wellness* is that it breaks down heart health into manageable, easy-to-follow weekly steps that incorporate key aspects of health and wellness, like the importance of a healthy diet, relaxation/meditation, and exercise to heal the heart and keep it beating strong."

—J.R., Pueblo, Colorado

HEART
to Soul
CARDIAC WELLNESS

AN INSPIRING PLAN TO
HOLISTICALLY PREVENT
AND RECOVER FROM
HEART DISEASE

MARY YUTER, RN, CCRN

WITH BERNICE PASS-STERN, MS, MED

This book is dedicated to my patients and their families.

THEY TAUGHT ME HOW TO APPRECIATE THE LOVE AND MEANING OF LIFE MORE THAN ANY TEXTBOOK COULD. THANK YOU FOR ALLOWING ME TO BE A PART OF YOUR LIFE STORIES LIVED WITH SUCH GRACE.

Cover and interior design by Domini Dragoone • dominidragoone.com
Editorial services provided by Jill Rothenberg • jillrothenberg.com
Author photo © Laura Jane Brett • laurajanebrettphotography.com
Cover images: SamPosnick/iStock, NicoOlay/iStock

ISBN (print): 978-1-7361435-9-9
ISBN (ebook): 978-1-7361435-4-4

For large or bulk orders, please email hearttosoulcw@gmail.com

CONTENTS

FOREWORD

It was an ordinary Tuesday in early March of 2020. But it would soon become unforgettable. I was about to kick off the afternoon session at the 3rd Annual Northwell Heart Failure Therapies Conference at the Donald and Barbara Zucker Medical School in Long Island, New York, as a featured speaker to a group of cardiac physicians and nurses. My assignment was to relate my patient experience as the recipient of a Left Ventricular Assist Device (LVAD) in this relatively new Heart Failure and Heart Transplant Center, the first of its kind on Long Island.

While I was already an experienced public speaker on dental disease and more recently on congestive heart failure and the multitude of issues related to that subject, I found myself feeling particularly proud and grateful to be there, at that moment, having come from the depths of hopelessness and five life-saving heart operations. At around noon, an hour before I was to go on, I was approached by a genuinely warm and kind woman, a stranger who seemed to know exactly why I was there. Her name was Mary Yuter, a former cardiac ICU registered nurse who had recently started her own cardiac wellness business, www.hearttosoulcw.com. It was immediately obvious to me that this was not the kind of person you meet every day. Mary could not have been kinder and more generous to both me and my wife as we ambled through the academic theatre awaiting my turn to take the stage. We briefly told Mary about our incredible experiences over the past year, mine as a heart failure patient and my wife's as my newly anointed caregiver. She asked that we keep in touch, and my instincts told me to follow through on that promise.

Mary and I began to meet regularly, online, as the COVID-19 pandemic began to ravage the world. We shared ideas about how we and others can be better healthcare providers and how we can make the experience of being a patient with heart disease more meaningful, more informed, and more hopeful. Mary's intelligence, insight, and positive outlook was unlike anything that I had ever encountered. Her encyclopedic knowledge of heart health and her thirst for learning was both inspiring and exciting, giving me even more hope than I already had as a heart failure patient who, to this point, had achieved a stunning recovery.

Mary's book, *Heart to Soul Cardiac Wellness*, is the most ambitious, most complete, most optimistic guide for anyone wanting to avoid heart disease, or to heal from a recent bout with heart disease, that I have ever read. Mary's firsthand experience treating the most seriously affected cardiac patients, and her passion for wanting to share her knowledge about what it takes to stay alive and truly live in the face of heart disease, make her the perfect mentor and companion in your journey toward better health.

Now I know that I could have probably done a better job of taking care of my heart in the twenty-two years that I have battled heart disease. Perhaps I was more focused on maintaining my practice as a cosmetic and restorative dentist, keeping my marriage (40 years this year!) strong, and raising my two sons. And I was certainly proud of these accomplishments. Wouldn't it have been great to have a guide to show me exactly what to do in order to possibly avoid developing Congestive Heart Failure? What should I have eaten? How should I have exercised? How should I have relaxed after a stressful day?

For the people who are lucky enough to be reading this book, *you* now have the guide I have been fortunate enough to have. You have the guide who will help support you in a clear, concise and encouraging manner, to avoid heart disease and to lessen the chance of repeated heart disease in the case that, like me, you have already had your heart's "moment of awakening."

Besides the lessons that you will learn to help avoid becoming sick or getting sick again, by following the lessons in this book, you will learn to "adapt to change." In fact, your "new life" might be even better than your "old life"! Now, it may not be easy, as Mary points out in this book. But... nothing worth doing is easy! You will learn things about yourself that you never knew. You will learn how your heart and the rest of your body works. It's like when I was learning to walk again after I came home from the hospital; my physical therapist taught me that walking was more about breathing correctly than anything else. I never knew that. Imagine learning not only all about how your body works, but how *you* can be the supervisor of the whole operation.

I have always taught my students, audience members, and fellow healthcare providers to show gratitude toward those who might have contributed to their education and success. In this book, Mary shows us that gratitude not only serves others but also serves ourselves. Expressing gratitude for the things and people around us that allow us to continue to thrive actually serves to calm ourselves in the face of the unknown and in the face of necessary change.

Now for most of us mere mortals, much is being asked here. Changing the way we cook, eat, sleep, exercise and even think is certainly a pretty steep mountain to climb. However, *Heart to Soul Cardiac Wellness* will serve as your "mountain climbing team." While I say in my presentations, "YOU are the most important part of your recovery," *you* are certainly not alone in this new challenge now that you have found your new companion.

I am grateful to have met Mary Yuter when I did. It was at exactly the right time for me. Take this gradual, inspiring, life-changing journey with Mary through *Heart to Soul Cardiac Wellness*. Get ready for your new informative, exciting and wonderful life!

Have a safe and hopeful journey.

—Gary C. Sherman, D.M.D., Heart Failure Thriver
   Dentist, Professional Speaker on Congestive Heart Failure,
   Amateur Golfer, Husband and Dad

PART ONE

YOUR HARD WORK *and effort* WILL NOT GO *unrewarded.*

Welcome

TO HEART TO SOUL CARDIAC WELLNESS

I wrote *Heart to Soul Cardiac Wellness* to help you become a Cardiac Thriver and to give survivors of a cardiac event hope.

The information in *Heart to Soul Cardiac Wellness* will help you as you learn how to navigate your heart-healthy life. It will teach you how to prevent heart disease, recover from a heart attack, and to prepare for, or recuperate from a cardiac event such as open-heart surgery. In short, this book will take your hand and help you on your way to better health.

Heart to Soul Cardiac Wellness will provide you with peace of mind because here you have a plan, with knowledge and tools you can easily put into daily practice. You will be empowered to become the guardian of your health. Most importantly, you can have hope in knowing that you can start now, today, wherever you are on your quest for heart health, wellness, and recovery, and reap the benefits of a new lifestyle going forward.

As a cardiac ICU (Intensive Care Unit) nurse in New York City, in the premier award-winning cardiac care unit (CCU) of the oldest public hospital in the United States, I took care of people just like you. They did not understand why and how they got so sick, or what they could do to change and improve their health. Unfortunately, medical doctors and nurses are not trained in alternative healing options which complement Western medicine. When used together, the combination of both healing modalities can dramatically improve a patient's health, rather than one option alone. In the culture of our *reactive* "sick-care" system (instead of *proactive, preventive* healthcare), doctors and nurses do not have the time to speak to their patients about how best to prevent disease. It is impossible to do, if they only have 10–15 minutes to see a patient while also completing the medical charting for that visit, calling in any prescriptions and getting updates from the patient on any changes to their health, and then addressing those new health issues as well.

Heart patients, like those who have had heart attacks, heart failure, pacemaker implants, ablations, or post open-heart surgery, get readmitted to the hospital because they never made lifestyle changes (they never knew to do so), so they got sicker. Think about it: If a person gets sick from something they were doing, and this is not corrected, they will continue to be sick because the *cause* of their illness has not been addressed.

"YOU CAN'T GO BACK AND CHANGE THE BEGINNING, BUT YOU CAN START WHERE YOU ARE AND CHANGE THE ENDING."
—**C.S. LEWIS,** writer

Here, I share everything I ever wanted to tell my patients about how to course correct their lifestyle in order to improve their heart health and overall wellness. I did not have the opportunity to do so in the very short amount of time I had with a patient. Sadly, at the time of their hospital discharge, my patients went home with only a bag of medications, post-op wound care instructions, and a follow-up visit scheduled, after a life-altering medical emergency such as open-heart surgery or a heart attack, without a comprehensive plan or resources to help them make effective changes to heal and regain their health. These patients left the hospital and walked off into an abyss of fear, without any solid plan or information to help them in recovery.

These patients inspired me to create this book for *you*; it will serve as your wellness and recovery safety net. You now have a plan in these pages so you don't fall into an abyss of fear. You will feel confident with your plan, at peace, and feel nurtured because you are supported. You will be empowered to take charge of your health and wellness with the knowledge you will gain. You will learn a lot.

"BEFORE YOU HEAL SOMEONE, ASK HIM IF HE IS WILLING TO GIVE UP THE THINGS THAT MADE HIM SICK."

—HIPPOCRATES, "The Father of Medicine"

Are you ready to give up things that are making you sick so you can make room to receive the things that will help you get well?

This book will show you what makes us sick and how you can make changes to prevent illness. It will also help heal your heart so you can live a healthier life. The information presented here serves as a preventative measure against heart disease by using weekly, easy-to-follow steps to improve heart health, which leads to overall well-being. There are segments of this nine-week program that focus on nutrition and why what we eat matters, self-care, exercise, friendships and the importance of family and social connection, all with the goal of providing the tools and support you need to take proactive control of your health and prevent disease.

> This book is not a substitute for medical advice, diagnosis or treatment. This book is not to be used in place of your doctor's medical plan for you. The information in this book is meant to complement your doctor's medical plan. Always seek the advice of your physician with any questions you have regarding a medical condition, and before undertaking any diet, dietary supplement, exercise, or other health program.
>
> The information presented in this book is based on my professional experience. I encourage you to supplement what is presented in this book with your own research, as the science of health and wellness is constantly changing.

SO—WITH THAT, HERE WE GO!
LET'S BEGIN BY TALKING ABOUT HEART DISEASE.

Heart disease has been the number one cause of death in the United States for decades, killing more people every year than *all cancers combined*, yet it is largely preventable.

The Centers for Disease Control and Prevention report that about 655,000 Americans die of heart disease every year. That translates to 1 in every 4 deaths resulting from heart disease.

The American Heart Association states that each year, there are about 335,000 recurrent heart attacks. Of the survivors of a first heart attack, 1 in 5 people will have a second heart attack within five years; many of them not surviving a second heart attack. These people may not have had to suffer or die and their heart disease could possibly have been prevented.

> **If heart disease is the number one cause of death in the United States—shouldn't heart disease be considered a national health emergency?**

IT'S NOT. WHY NOT?

Well, sick people make money for others in their need for, and use of costly medications, medical appointments, tests, procedures, operations, and hospitalizations. Healthy people, not so much, right?

If heart disease is preventable, then why are so many people dying of it? Why do so many people say they have a "family history" of heart disease? What can we do to change this so we don't become yet another statistic?

I wrote this book to answer these questions, to bring awareness to this disease process, and to offer a plan of help and hope so we can collectively heal and improve our heart health together. Heart disease won't be the number one cause of death anymore if we all take care of our health.

As a nurse, many people I cared for were readmitted to the hospital in far worse shape than they were during their prior admission. Some of the patients I took care of never knew that day would be the last time they saw their family, their dog or cat, their home, or that they had turned their key to lock their front door for the very last time. One patient was readmitted a year to the date of his first admission, in the same room, with me again as his nurse. I couldn't believe it when I saw his name on the monitor and I thought it must be a person with the same name, until I entered the room and saw his wife sitting at the bedside. Then I recognized the unforgettable sleeve tattoo on his arm, which was lying limply on the bed because he was sedated, on multiple life-saving intravenous drip medications, and on several machines for life support. He had not altered the things that made him sick enough for his first hospital admission, so he got critically ill again. He is lucky because he was granted another opportunity in his life to make positive health and lifestyle changes. He now has a pacemaker and a defibrillator implanted in his chest. Many patients were never this lucky because their illness and loss of a vibrant life were preventable.

SO, WHAT IS GOING ON?
WHY ARE SO MANY PEOPLE SICK WITH HEART DISEASE?

Well, in the hospital, I could almost recite what the night nurse was going to tell me about the patient I was about to receive from him or her during the 7:00 a.m. shift change. The patient would inevitably have one, if not all three of the following health issues, which greatly contribute to cardiac disease and chronic illness: Hypertension, (high blood pressure) Hyperlipidemia, (high cholesterol and fats) and Type 2 diabetes, (high blood sugar). I call these three the "Cardiac Bermuda Triangle" because if no intervention is done, you can get caught up in this triangle of illness. Preventing these diseases is key to avoiding heart disease, our country's number one cause of death. The good news is that these health issues can be reversible. The following nine-week journey with me will have you thinking differently about your food, your wellness, and your health. This program will bring you hope and positivity because now you have a plan to optimize your health against heart disease. If you already have any heart disease, or have had an event such as a heart attack, or open-heart surgery, or have ongoing heart failure, I want you to know that there is hope for you to feel better, improve your health, and have the lab results to prove it!

LET'S BEGIN OUR JOURNEY BY HONORING YOU.

You may have asked yourself these questions: "What can I do to optimize my health?" "Where do I start?" "What can I do so that I won't get sick again?" I understand your concerns and I hear you. You are *definitely* in the right spot. Week by week, you will build on your knowledge, which will empower you to make health and lifestyle changes that will result in positive effects that you can see and feel in your overall physical and emotional health. The way I am writing each page is as if I am talking to you, getting you ready to face a new beginning in your life. I also had in mind the family member or support person who was with you, scared, yet wanting to help you make health changes, yet not knowing how.

You are not alone in your healing and wellness journey. There are other people just like you starting this journey as well. It is no coincidence you are holding this book in your hands. *Heart to Soul Cardiac Wellness* was brought into your life to help you at the right time and it will positively change your life if you work with it daily as your coach and friend.

As you begin this book, I invite you to join me and other Cardiac Thrivers like you in a weekly on-line live class as we step through this book together. As a *Heart to Soul Cardiac Wellness* community, we support each other in our work, have discussions on pertinent topics, set goals and offer assistance to one another week by week. You may also want to join the group after you have completed this book to reinforce your learning and to gather tips and information from other people traveling on your wellness path. Please see the website www.hearttosoulcw.com for further information and to sign up for classes. There you will find classes for recovery after a heart attack, preparing for and recuperating from heart surgery, and best of all, your spouse/partner/caregiver can attend class together with you.

Wherever you are on your heart health journey, it's important to know that you are not alone. In addition to others on this path with you, your ultimate life accountability partner on this journey is the person you see in your bathroom mirror each day. Let's make that person in the mirror proud. Give yourself a full, all-in commitment with your book and you will see a positive change in the person who looks back at you from the mirror.

LITTLE BY LITTLE, SMALL ACTIONS ADD UP TO BECOME HUGE ACCOMPLISHMENTS OVER TIME.

You must be committed to changing your lifestyle and your behavior in order to change your health. Your success is 100 percent up to you. You have to own it. Like any goal in life, you have to want it first. Do you want to be healthier? Are you ready to give up the things that are making you sick so you have the room in your life to get healthier? Are you ready to learn? Do you want to get a sparkle back into your eyes and feel vibrant in living your life more fully? If you answered "Yes!" to these past questions, then let's move on. We have work to do!

How to Use
YOUR BOOK TO GET THE BEST OUT OF IT

Although it may be tempting to skip over sections that don't seem to reflect your experience, it is important to take the chapters in order. Information in the chapters builds in steps as you go along. Something you read may not seem relevant to you today, but could be important for you (or a loved one) later on. We may be confronted with topics or information we might not want to see or hear, but it's often the case that we can't make important life changes if we don't have full information or know how to address what we are doing wrong or what we can improve.

Topics have been organized to serve as building blocks of foundational information expanded into additional concepts in subsequent chapters. The chapters are structured a week apart so that you can take your time to absorb the content and make small lifestyle improvements each week. Week by week, before you know it, you will have made big enhancements to your life from these changes as you take over the driver's seat in your health. It will be like a weekly tune-up for your body and mind, Heart to Soul!

An important exception is for those who are scheduled to have cardiac surgery, who should first read the chapter titled *Pre-Op: Preparing For Your Heart Surgery* and then read the chapter titled: *Post-Op: Recovering From Your Heart Surgery*.

Understanding the surgery and recovery processes can help to ease your fear because you will understand the "hows" and "whys" of what is going on during your hospital stay. You will enter your surgery and your hospital visit with knowledge so you can anticipate what to expect. It is highly recommended that your partner, caregiver, or spouse read Part Three of this book as it will inform their understanding of the surgery process and how they can support you better while caring for themselves, too.

PRO TIP: Regardless of whether you have had heart surgery, there are additional takeaways in the Pre-op and Post-op sections that could help you or a loved one to prepare for and recover from any type of surgery.

Your *Heart to Soul Cardiac Wellness* book will be your nurturing partner for the next 66 days, a week at a time to help you start your wellness journey. Researchers have found that it takes an average of 66 days to make a behavior change that can then turn into a permanent habit, as reported in "How are habits formed: Modeling habit formation in the real world," by Phillippa Lally and colleagues in the October 2010 issue of the *European Journal of Social Psychology*. When we keep doing something consistently we can form a new "good" habit, which can lead to a lifestyle change, resulting in a positive impact to our health.

HEART TO SOUL CARDIAC WELLNESS, WEEK BY WEEK

Here's the plan: You will have a weekly chapter to read with a helpful exercise to help you absorb and apply what you have just read. This is usually a recommendation to watch a movie or video clip online or to complete a reading, all of which reinforce your learning of the chapter content for the week. Week by week, little adjustments you make as a result of what you have learned in the chapter content will add up to form big powerful changes for your health.

This book is presented in an interactive format and it encourages your participation as its team member on "Team YOU!" In between chapters, while you are absorbing the weekly chapter reading, you will check in with your book to complete your daily activities for each day in your journal.

The daily journal guides you to reflect on interactive prompts such as writing down three things you are grateful for that day, then to record your thoughts in writing. Writing can seem scary at first, but it is a useful tool. Don't worry about how it sounds or if it's grammatically correct or even in full sentences. The act of writing it down makes your commitment to heart health concrete. In the journal, you will be reinforcing your new daily routines, starting each day with breath work and a meditation, and ending each day with a gratitude reflection. In a way, the journal is your guide, your prompt, and your encouragement. Once you have started using the tools in this book, you will understand that before, it might have been as if you were driving a car all over the road. Now, you have a map for each day, and a plan for where you are going.

After each week of journaling and assignment completion, you can advance to the next chapter, then complete the corresponding exercises and daily journaling through the end of that week, until before you know it, you are done. In a nutshell: read a chapter a week, enjoy your "homework assignments," and complete a week's worth of thoughtful journaling. Our time together will go quickly as we work on these steps toward not only heart health but by creating your best life. I am really excited for you!

> **PRO TIP**: Please set aside uninterrupted quality time to enable you to devote mindful attention as you work with your book.

GRAPHS

There is nothing like a visual aid! By plotting your daily self-reported health scores on a graph, you will visually see your progress. You will document your overall feeling of wellness in your body and mind, from a low of 1 "We have work to do!" to a top "I feel fantastic!" score of 10 on your daily wellness graphs. You will record your daily weight on the daily weight "Weighing In" graph.

Heart to Soul Cardiac Wellness includes a graph to plot your daily pre-breakfast morning glucose level before you eat or drink anything, should you be a diabetic.

At the end of the 66-day journey, when you look at these graphs that have been compiled from your daily recordings, you will see how your wellness score has gone up and your morning glucose trend (if diabetic) has gone down. You will be able to track your lab values and vital signs to see the results of the improvements you have made, from baseline starting point to completion of the 9-week program. By making the life changes outlined, you may feel better; your labs and vital signs may improve, and you may even be able to decrease, or even stop taking some medications, only with your doctor's oversight. How would that feel to you?

> **NOTE:** The information in this book is not meant to take the place of your doctor's medical plan for you. Your doctor will be the one to make any medication or dosage alterations. *Do NOT* change the way you take your medications or begin any exercise program without first seeing and consulting with your doctor.

Your doctor is an important part of your journey. Take your book with you to your doctor so you can put your baseline labs into the spaces provided below. Share the book with your doctor, because they may not have seen it or even be aware of it… yet! Your doctor's office can help you with your health information that they have on record and it will only take a minute or two to complete. You will record and trend your baseline lab results and information such as vital signs and weight from the start of the book to completion. Don't worry if you don't have a scale at home to record your daily weight; how your clothes fit and how you feel in them will also tell you how you are doing.

The key aspect of your journey to heart wellness is in your mindset. Are you ready to be open to new ideas about optimizing your physical, mental, and spiritual health? Are you ready to shift your mindset to one of positivity and success? Are you ready to change your life by trying new things that will help you form a healthy lifestyle and especially to prevent cardiac events and instead optimize both heart health and your overall well-being? Are you ready to give up foods and old lifestyle habits that are making you sick and further, that can damage your heart? Are you ready to say, "I *could* do that, but I chose *not to*, because it is not good for me"?

To be successful, the answers to those questions need to be an all-in **YES!**

Here are some useful and empowering mantras that can accompany you throughout your journey:

YES, I can do this!

YES, I want to change my health!

YES, I want to feel vibrant and healthy!

YES, I want to feel good and have sparkle in my eyes!

Believe it. Believe in yourself. Get fired up! You are on the way to empowering yourself and improving your heart and general health.

"THE MOST IMPORTANT THING IS YOU
MUST PUT EVERYBODY ON NOTICE THAT
YOU'RE HERE AND YOU ARE FOR REAL."
—KOBE BRYANT, professional NBA player

Following is an accountability agreement that affirms this commitment you are making for yourself for 66 days, and likely, beyond those days and on a new, heart-healthy path! It will lead to you looking in the mirror at the end of each of those 66 days and on into the future, so you can say "I did my best. I am proud of myself. I will continue to get better each day!"

Remember how tomorrow will feel by something you did today, especially if you struggled to do it. If you have a setback, take stock of where you went off course, and get back on the heart health trail. Take the pressure off of yourself. Receive what you can and do what you are able to, to make this a growth challenge, not a chore. There is no blame and there is no shame. Change is really difficult, especially when we are so used to doing something a certain way. It is downright hard to shift out of old patterns. Make peace with yourself so that you can proceed forward with loving kindness on your *Heart to Soul Cardiac Wellness* adventure. Even a little progress forward is still progress. Honor your progression forward on your health journey with compassionate compliance for yourself. You are supported and nurtured. Taking it all in, one day at a time, will get you to a place of health and well-being that forms a lifetime of new lifestyle habits.

"A STUMBLING BLOCK TO THE PESSIMIST IS A
STEPPING STONE TO THE OPTIMIST."

— **ELEANOR ROOSEVELT,** former First Lady of the United States, activist

---

MY HEART TO SOUL CARDIAC WELLNESS ACCOUNTABILITY AGREEMENT

This is an agreement with myself to know that I am worthy of receiving the information in my *Heart to Soul Cardiac Wellness* book. I will take this information and use the tools I receive every day for 66 days. I will improve my lab values, my glucose levels (if diabetic) and my health. I will feel better. I will make the changes needed in my life in order for this to happen. I will be open to new ways of healing that will complement my physician's medical plan for me. I will expand my horizons by doing so. I look forward to learning new things to improve my health.

I will complete my *Heart to Soul Cardiac Wellness* plan in 66 days. I will have compassionate compliance with myself because I know it may not be easy.

Hard work is not easy, but I know my work efforts will have positive results for me. I know I am supported on my health journey with this book.

I will complete my *Heart to Soul Cardiac Wellness* book successfully. I will change my health. I will feel better. I will welcome change so I may become an example for others. I will become my best version of myself.

Please sign below to confirm your agreement with yourself.

I, _____
feel gratitude because I know all of this to be true.

Today's date is:

_____

66 Days from now, the date will be:

_____

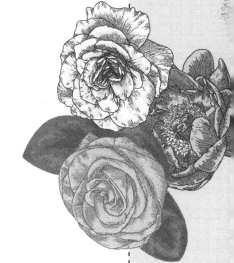

You've got this! Now let's begin our *Heart to Soul Cardiac Wellness* journey together! Are you ready? **Let's go!**

"WHEN ONE DOOR CLOSES, ANOTHER OPENS; BUT WE OFTEN LOOK SO LONG AND SO REGRETFULLY UPON THE CLOSED DOOR THAT WE DO NOT SEE THE ONE WHICH WAS OPENED FOR US."

—ALEXANDER GRAHAM BELL, Scottish-born inventor, scientist, engineer

----

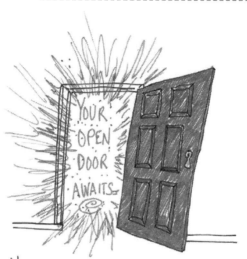

You are always just one decision away from walking through the open door of your divine destiny. Sometimes you cannot see it is a door, but it's always there... awaiting you. The door is only locked if you think it is. Of course, you may not want to walk through. It might mean changing your friends, your habits, your identity & your place here. There's no lock on the door. No ogre or guardian... The limit is only how much you are willing to step fully to the other side. Realizing things will never be the same again. You cannot 'undo' this particular decision, which is why so many choose to knock or shuffle around the entrance hoping for a peek. That's not the way it works. You surrender fully and let go of fear... drop the stories holding you back from truly knowing what's on the other side.

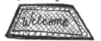

Used with permission from Yanik Silver, creator of the *Cosmic Journal*.

YOUR
Personal
CHEMISTRY SET

It's not necessarily your genetics that causes disease. It's what is on the end of your fork that is bringing you one step closer either to illness or wellness. It's not necessarily your DNA, it's your dinner that leads you closer to heart health or further away from it. The bottom line: What you are eating and drinking can make you sick.

What is in our DNA is in part our culture regarding food. You may have a "family history" of heart disease but that may be due to your "family history" of eating patterns. We have culturally assimilated eating certain foods going back through generations. Our ancestors have died from cardiac disease or other chronic diseases because of their cultural food consumption. My Italian friend said "You can't separate me from my mozzarella!" Well, a scalpel might have to one day.

Before I gave it up for my health, I used to love the taste of bacon, and I came to find out that my ancestors were not only pig farmers, they were also cattle ranchers. My family members ate pork and beef daily. As a result, I have a family history of many types of cancers. I share this with you because the things we are routinely eating are working against us, causing disease. This can cause tremendous strain on our heart and additional burden to the body as it works so hard to constantly right itself.

In the pages that follow, we will explore this in depth. You will learn what to do to protect yourself and help ease the work required of your heart and body. To begin, we will look at how the lifestyle changes we make can positively affect us, beginning with our lab work—your personal chemistry set.

LET'S SEE WHERE WE ARE NOW: YOUR BASELINE (STARTING) LABS

You cannot see heart disease on the outside of a person. Our unique blood lab values, for instance cholesterol or A1c, tell a big part of the story of our health. We each have our own personal chemistry set, with values unique to us, and we are able to change those values to optimize them by how we treat our bodies. Humans have a range of each lab value that we fall into as a "normal" range. Below, you are going to track your baseline, or initial labs, before we start our 66 days together. This is your initial reference point to see how far you have come and in what areas you need to further continue your work or maintain your values. You will need to get your end of program lab values at the conclusion of the 66 days. Tracking your progress daily will allow you over time to see positive changes in your lab values and in your health.

Your provider or insurance may not cover the full scope of the labs, so please verify which lab tests are covered, and get any lab work that you can under your plan. **Non-standard labs may require additional charges, and it is okay if you cannot get all the labs due to charges.** Let's work with what labs you can get at this time. If you do not have insurance now, and cannot get the blood tests, that is ok. You can still make positive progress in your health. When you can get blood tests, the labs you need are listed below.

> **NOTE: Your bloodwork should be scheduled for and taken in the morning after fasting all night and before you eat anything in the morning.** A little water is okay and it is a good idea to bring healthy snacks like fruit with you to eat immediately after your blood draw to avoid hypoglycemia, (low blood sugar) which can make you feel shaky, cold, and sweaty.

LAB VALUES

Please note: "normal" or "ideal" value ranges may vary slightly, depending on the lab, institution, or medical provider.

	Baseline	End of Program	Ideal
HDL			>50
LDL			<100
Cholesterol			<200
Triglycerides			<150
Total Chol/HDL			<3.5
Lipoprotein (a)			<30
TMAO			<6.2

The above labs are your levels of lipids or fats in the blood and also provide information regarding cardiac disease risk. HDL is the "good" cholesterol that helps to remove the LDL, or "bad" cholesterol, from your blood vessels.

	Baseline	End of Program	Ideal
Cortisol (am)			4–22
C reactive protein			<8
Sed rate			<30

The labs above are inflammatory markers that show how much inflammation there is in the body. Inflammation is good when the body responds to an acute (new) localized wound—like putting out a fire in the toaster oven. Inflammation is not good when the body has a chronic (ongoing) fire in the whole house.

Below are standard labs for your "blood chemistry," the Complete Blood Count and the Basic Metabolic tests. These values are good to note baseline to highlight any outliers with your physician, as there are many components to each of these tests. You will not need to fill in the values for Complete Blood Count and Basic Metabolic tests, however, you should review these results with your doctor for any irregularities.

	Baseline	End of Program
Complete Blood Count	Irregularities?	Resolved?
Basic Metabolic	Irregularities?	Resolved?

The following labs are vitamins and amino acids that we need to monitor in our body. Many people are deficient in these, which impedes the body's ability to function optimally.

	Baseline	End of Program	Ideal
Vitamin B12			200–1100
Vitamin D			30–100
Omega 3			>3.2

	Baseline	End of Program	Ideal
Folate			>5.4
Homocysteine			<10.4

High Homocysteine amino acid levels are related to vitamin deficiency, and they also serve as a cardiac disease indicator.

	Baseline	End of Program	Ideal
Fasting glucose			<85
A1c			<5.7

A1c is the way your body uses glucose over a three-month period by looking at the blood cells, similarly to looking at the rings of wood in a tree. A high A1c level is an indicator of diabetes.

LET'S LOOK AT YOUR VITAL STATISTICS NOW.

	Baseline	End of Program	Ideal
Blood Pressure			120/80
Heart rate			60–100
Weight			
Height			
BMI*			18.5–24.8

*BMI, your Body Mass Index, measures how healthy your weight is in relation to your height. BMI serves as a tool for assessing your risk for weight related health problems.

> **PRO TIP**: There are calculators online to help you obtain your BMI (Body Mass Index) such as NHLBI.NIH.GOV which will calculate your BMI in American measurement units.

Let's explore some more about where you are in your health journey now. Sometimes the act of sitting and processing these questions may bring about an "Ah-ha!" moment, perhaps causing you to realize something about yourself that you never have before.

	Baseline	End of Program	Ideal
On a score of 1–100%, how do you feel today?			90–100%
Do you smoke?	Yes / No	Yes / No	No
(Males) Erectile Dysfunction?	Yes / No	Yes / No	No

What are your other health diagnoses and health challenges?

Where are you now in your overall health? Where do you want to be?

How do you want to feel?

ALLERGIES

Are you wearing an allergy alert bracelet? If not, you may consider getting one to wear. List your allergies below in the space provided.

Allergic to:	Reaction:

Allergic to:	Reaction:

Allergic to:	Reaction:

FALL RISK

Do you wear a fall alert necklace? If you do opt to get one, look for one that doesn't solely rely on you pressing the button to activate the notification process that you had a fall. There are fall alert necklaces that perform time and motion studies that can possibly tell if you fell, (an example is if you fainted) and you were not able to press the button. These functions may be a little more expensive, but the peace of mind they offer are worth that extra layer of protection.

STRESSORS

What are the primary stressors that you have in your life? Do you have any additional stressors out of the ordinary, such as a recent death in the family, job loss, child care or elder care concerns, or marital problems?

MEDICATIONS

List what medications you are taking and why you are taking them, below. **Put a dated copy of your medications, dosage and how often you take the medication in your wallet, so in the event emergency personnel need this information, it is available.** Tell your family about this list as well. Give your family members a copy of your medication list. This list will need to be continuously updated and distributed any time you have a medication change.

Date on medication:	*(month/day/year)*
Name of medication:	*(Medication XYZ)*
Baseline dosage:	25mg, twice a day, at 9:00 am and 9:00 pm
Reason(s) for taking:	I am taking Medication XYZ because I had a heart attack, and I have high blood pressure and I need to keep my blood pressure down to help my heart pump easier.
Ending dosage:	

Note: The field marked "Ending dosage" will be filled in upon completion of your 66 days.

If you are not sure what the medications are used to treat or why you are taking the medications, ask your doctor. **Please specify medication dosage information such as micrograms, milligrams, or grams, or units and type for insulin.**

Date on medication:	
Name of medication:	
Baseline dosage:	
Reason(s) for taking:	
Ending dosage:	

Date on medication:	
Name of medication:	
Baseline dosage:	
Reason(s) for taking:	
Ending dosage:	

Date on medication:	
Name of medication:	
Baseline dosage:	
Reason(s) for taking:	
Ending dosage:	

Date on medication:	
Name of medication:	
Baseline dosage:	
Reason(s) for taking:	
Ending dosage:	

Date on medication:	
Name of medication:	
Baseline dosage:	
Reason(s) for taking:	
Ending dosage:	

Date on medication:	
Name of medication:	
Baseline dosage:	
Reason(s) for taking:	
Ending dosage:	

Date on medication:	
Name of medication:	
Baseline dosage:	
Reason(s) for taking:	
Ending dosage:	

Date on medication:	
Name of medication:	
Baseline dosage:	
Reason(s) for taking:	
Ending dosage:	

Date on medication:	
Name of medication:	
Baseline dosage:	
Reason(s) for taking:	
Ending dosage:	

Date on medication:	
Name of medication:	
Baseline dosage:	
Reason(s) for taking:	
Ending dosage:	

Date on medication:	
Name of medication:	
Baseline dosage:	
Reason(s) for taking:	
Ending dosage:	

Date on medication:	
Name of medication:	
Baseline dosage:	
Reason(s) for taking:	
Ending dosage:	

Date on medication:	
Name of medication:	
Baseline dosage:	
Reason(s) for taking:	
Ending dosage:	

WEIGHT IN POUNDS

110 120 130 140 150 160 170 180 190 200 210 220 230 240 250 260 270 280 290 300 310 320 330

DAY OF PROGRAM

1
2
3
4
5
6
7
8
9
10
11
12
13
14
15
16
17
18
19
20
21
22
23
24
25
26
27
28
29
30

110 120 130 140 150 160 170 180 190 200 210 220 230 240 250 260 270 280 290 300 310 320 330

31
32
33
34
35
36
37
38
39
40
41
42
43
44
45
46
47
48
49
50
51
52
53
54
55
56
57
58
59
60
61
62
63
64
65
66

DAILY WELLNESS TRACKER: How are you feeling today on a scale of 1–10? Plot it on this graph! If you aren't happy with how you feel, what can you do today so that you feel better tomorrow?.

	1	2	3	4	5	6	7	8	9	10

DAY OF PROGRAM

1
2
3
4
5
6
7
8
9
10
11
12
13
14
15
16
17
18
19
20
21
22
23
24
25
26
27
28
29
30

	1	2	3	4	5	6	7	8	9	10
31										
32										
33										
34										
35										
36										
37										
38										
39										
40										
41										
42										
43										
44										
45										
46										
47										
48										
49										
50										
51										
52										
53										
54										
55										
56										
57										
58										
59										
60										
61										
62										
63										
64										
65										
66										

MORNING GLUCOSE LEVEL

	100	110	120	130	140	150	160	170	180	190	200	210	220	230	240	250+

DAY OF PROGRAM

1
2
3
4
5
6
7
8
9
10
11
12
13
14
15
16
17
18
19
20
21
22
23
24
25
26
27
28
29
30

	100	110	120	130	140	150	160	170	180	190	200	210	220	230	240	250+
31																
32																
33																
34																
35																
36																
37																
38																
39																
40																
41																
42																
43																
44																
45																
46																
47																
48																
49																
50																
51																
52																
53																
54																
55																
56																
57																
58																
59																
60																
61																
62																
63																
64																
65																
66																

PART TWO

TURN
the beat
AROUND!

Week 1:
SELF-CARE FOR YOU IS SELF-CARE FOR ALL

By taking care of yourself, you will be able to show up to be fully present for your family, your friends, your work and in short, your life. By showing others that you care about yourself, you are setting an example of a positive intention for health. This isn't about taking a bath and calling it self-care; there is more to it than that. I want to ease your worries about getting sick or sick *again*, because you will be empowered to take the best care of your body.

SO… WHAT DO I MEAN BY "SELF-CARE?"

Let's start by looking at how you begin your day. For most people, they get up because an alarm barked them out of bed, their feet hit the floor, they guzzle down sweetened coffee or maybe even a soda or an energy drink and quickly eat a sugary breakfast item as they push themselves out the door. If at home, they may be in "sloth-mode" on the couch, pushing the buttons on the TV remote, waiting to see what the day brings to them. One of the first things they do is look at their phone.

Existing day to day is not a way to take charge of your life, or to max out each day to its fullest potential.

NOW, LET'S LOOK AT A DIFFERENT SCENARIO

Today's plan began the night before by looking at your calendar, checking-in on what plans and commitments you have, mentally preparing for what the day will look like and what you want to accomplish.

The alarm is set for an extra 15 minutes earlier. When the alarm clock goes off, you check-in with your body. How does it feel today? How do you feel overall? Do you have any areas that are cranky and need attention? With this extra few minutes of morning time, you do a series of deep breathing exercises, what I will refer to as breath work, to energize your cells and body. You then enjoy a 10-minute guided meditation to allow your mind to clear and to ground yourself to prepare you for whatever the day may bring. You create a mindful intention word for the day. You pick one word as your theme word for the day; *peace, gratitude, purpose, empathy, authenticity, compassion, generosity, knowledge, trust, openness, success, spirituality, enlightenment, ethics, release, healing, vibrant, integrity* and *contentment* are examples. You get mentally fired up about the possibilities of this new day before you. You are consciously aware that you have the gift of this day to spend and the opportunity of time that other people could only wish for. Imagine the person who is lying in bed, dying in hospice, wishing that despite your own obstacles, they would take your situation and make the best of it because it meant they were alive and had a chance.

The message here is: Today is a gift you were given to enjoy; that is why it is called the "present." Receive, honor, and enjoy each day.

"IF YOU LOVE LIFE, DON'T WASTE TIME, FOR
TIME IS WHAT LIFE IS MADE UP OF."

—BRUCE LEE, actor, martial artist, philosopher

The above scenarios reflect the difference between living your life with intention, making choices with your highest self in mind or living your life by passively existing. You have choices. You can choose to coast along, but that mode of living will not help you move forward in your life. Living with positivity, intention, and purpose takes energy and thoughtfulness, but with your efforts you will be presenting your best self to the world and most importantly, to your accountability partner in the bathroom mirror each day.

LIFE IS WHAT HAPPENS WHEN YOU ARE NOT LOOKING AT A SCREEN

Monitor how much time you can waste on social media. Make a pact with yourself to not use your phone the first half hour of each day so that *you* are in control of your energy and the day's direction. How much time do you spend each day on social media? Make a time budget to limit the time and stick to it, especially in the mindless scrolling that is so easy to get caught up in, yet doesn't add joy or benefits to your day. It is helpful to have set timeframes when you check and return email and social media so you don't get interrupted and distracted from something more important.

Ask yourself: "Is what I am doing helping me improve?" "Is this moving the needle forward in my life?" Instead of wasting time on social media or with any screen that isn't necessary for work or for your well-being, use this time to ensure you have set up your day well, and you have a plan and goals. Know that every day is a special occasion and celebrate accordingly. Use the good silverware or the good china or that special vase or wear your favorite outfit. Allow yourself to do things that bring you joy and support you.

"DON'T COUNT THE DAYS; MAKE THE DAYS COUNT."
—MUHAMMAD ALI, boxer, activist, philanthropist

BREATH WORK

Breath work? You may be asking yourself "Why are we talking about breathing—I am already breathing nicely!" Well, this may be true, however we can use breath techniques to feed our cells and increase our energy. Breath work is a secret wellness tool you can use anywhere, anytime.

A new ritual—one as easy as breathing—can become an important part of your self-care journey to better heart health and the new lifestyle that comes with it. This is a moment for you to stop, pause for a time in kindness to yourself, and to start your day in a thoughtful and healing manner. Taking time to pause by doing intentional breathing, followed by meditation, allows you the time to start your day in control and in a positive frame of mind for what lies ahead.

Here's how it works: Upon getting out of bed, after using the bathroom to relieve yourself, weighing yourself and recording your weight in your daily journal space, sit in an upright position, hands on lower belly, feet flat on the floor, spine straight. A chair is often the best place for this exercise. Close your eyes and take about five minutes of deep breaths slowly through your nose as follows:

As you breathe in and out through your nose, feel your hands on your belly moving with each breath. Think of a toddler, walking on the beach with their belly moving in and out. When we breathe from our belly, we expand the grape cluster-like air exchange sacs at the base of the lungs called the alveoli. Expanding our breath to the base engages our body in the relaxation response, stimulating the bodies large Vagus nerve to activate the "Rest and Digest" mode of our nervous system. Consider the reaction you have when someone has surprised you; you quickly inhale to your upper chest, which activates the "Fight or Flight" part of your nervous system. This upper chest type of breathing is not as relaxing or as fulfilling to your body as belly breathing. Belly breathing allows your diaphragm to move more fully, your lungs to expand optimally, and this pressure indirectly massages your abdomen and lymph nodes, positively affecting your circulation.

During your belly breaths, if thoughts come up, (and they will), mentally step back, notice you are having a thought; label it "thought" and let it go. Think of your thoughts as bubbles going by, rising into the air. Continue to focus on the inhale of belly breaths to the slow easy count of 4 and the exhale of 7. Inhale, feel the coolness of the air in your nostrils, exhale feeling the warmth of the air as it leaves your body. Inhale the nourishment the oxygen brings your body, exhale anything that does not serve you. Empower yourself with strength from each breath. You can experiment with your breath work, inhaling to the word "healthy," exhaling to the word "calm," or any combination of words that make you feel relaxed, centered, and grounded. You can also repeat your intention word for the day in your mind with each breath.

"Box Breathing," another breathing technique described below, is a great time-out tool to call upon if you feel stressed and want to take a little time to gather your thoughts and emotions. Dr. Mark Hyman, a leading functional medicine doctor and author of many health and wellness books, refers to this breath exercise as "Take 5" breathing, useful before meals to improve digestion and to actively relax.

If you do *not* suffer from shortness of breath, or any medical contraindications, you can try this simple "Box Breathing" technique for calming and centering, which adds on the mental visual creation of a box: Sit upright, spine straight, feet flat on the floor, hands on your thighs, palms down. First, take a slow deep belly breath in and out to center yourself. Notice how you feel before starting. Close your eyes. Breathe in slowly, filling your belly to the count of 5, hold for the count of 5, release your breath to the count of 5, hold for the count of 5.

As you do your box breathing, think of drawing a box, the inhale is the line going up, the hold after inhale is a line across to the right, the breath release is a line down, and the hold on your exhale is a line right to left. You have drawn an imaginary box. Do 5 rounds of box breathing. As you are taking these breaths in and out and drawing your imaginary line, you are doing a form of meditation. You can add on an affirming or empowering phrase with each breath, such as "I am safe" or "I am healing." Once you are done with your box breathing, notice how you feel. Has the way your body and mind feel changed since before you did the box breathing? Next time you are in line at the market or waiting somewhere, you can call upon this breath work tool to help you relax.

MEDITATION

The goal of meditation is to allow our minds to clear, to allow space for new thoughts and inspiration to come to us. You are the observer of yourself in meditation. Reread that last sentence. Yes—you are observing your thoughts. It is almost like two people are present, you and the observer of you. You have the power to observe yourself through your meditation rather than judge yourself. Meditation builds our "emotional immune system" allowing the space and time to check out and to focus on "being" instead of "doing" all the time. Meditation offers comfort and grounding, allowing you to be with yourself. If you can't be alone with yourself, then how can you expect others to be with you, right? You can engage in a moving meditation as well, almost like a stream of consciousness, like when doing an activity such as biking or running, and you "get in the zone." Think of meditation as being similar to when you clean out the refrigerator; then you have room for fresh groceries. Meditating in the morning helps you to clear out mental clutter, allowing you to approach your day with a calm, quiet mind. I encourage you to research different kinds of meditation styles to see which type you like. A nice way to begin your exploration is with a "Loving Kindness" meditation. Look for these online and see which person's voice resonates with you.

> **PRO TIP**: It is easy to fall asleep if you are lying down when meditating, so it is best to sit upright, feet on the floor, palms on your thighs. There are special meditations to help you sleep, and for sure you can enjoy those while lying down!

> **PRO TIP**: Meditation takes practice. Start with short meditations of 5 minutes or so, and add on to longer meditations as you feel you can and want to. It may be hard to start meditating right away in what seems like a *Star Wars* Jedi Master-like 20-minute practice, so take the pressure off of yourself and take it slow. After all, it is called a meditation "practice," not a meditation "perfect."

> **PRO TIP**: There are lots of free meditations you can try online. It may take you a few tries to find someone whose voice is appealing to you. Please see the meditation Apps and free meditation resources listed in your *Resource Boutique* in the back of your book.

> **PRO TIP**: Set a daily repeating chime to ring on your phone for a time that is convenient for you each day, as your "positivity check-in moment." This chime serves to remind you to take a few deep belly breaths, pausing to honor yourself with a daily moment of gratitude for your effort on your path to wellness.

GRATITUDE

To close each day, spend quiet time with yourself. Think of three things you are grateful for and write them down in the daily journal space provided in your book. If you have a spiritual practice, you can call forth your faith in gratitude. Even if today was a really bad day, your lungs were breathing for you, your heart was beating for you and you were here with the possibility of something new for you and *tomorrow is a fresh start*.

"WHEN I STARTED COUNTING MY BLESSINGS, MY WHOLE LIFE TURNED AROUND."

—WILLIE NELSON, country musician

Gratitude is important because you can only have one emotion at a time. You can choose a gratitude moment versus anger when triggered, by stepping back into self-awareness. By removing ourselves from the emotions of the moment, we allow ourselves the choice to see what life lesson we can learn. Negative emotions are our reaction to a loss of power. We allow them to trigger us. Learning to seek what the situation and emotions are teaching you can be so powerful and empowering.

Gratitude can shift our reflex from reacting in the moment to coming back to revisit our situation, calm us down, and shift our perspective for a moment. Gratitude allows your body to release the "feel good" happiness hormones serotonin and dopamine to your brain. The root cause of a negative emotion may need to be readdressed, but you now have an "escape button" from immediate reactivity by using your friend gratitude.

"WHEN I WAS 5 YEARS OLD, MY MOTHER ALWAYS TOLD ME THAT HAPPINESS WAS THE KEY TO LIFE. WHEN I WENT TO SCHOOL, THEY ASKED ME WHAT I WANTED TO BE WHEN I GREW UP. I WROTE DOWN 'HAPPY'. THEY TOLD ME I DIDN'T UNDERSTAND THE ASSIGNMENT, AND I TOLD THEM THEY DIDN'T UNDERSTAND LIFE."

—**JOHN LENNON,** musician, peace activist

WEEKLY HOMEWORK

(CHECK OFF WHEN COMPLETED)

☐ Watch the movie *Heal* (2017) about the bodies' innate capacity to heal itself when provided support.

☐ Watch the movie *What the Health* (2017) about the politics behind our food.

☐ Look up and research the lifestyle of people who live in the "Blue Zones." These healthy people live to be some of the oldest in the world due to their lifestyle. Why?

JOY & MEANING
JOURNAL PAGES

Make a list here of things that make you happy, or bring joy and meaning to your life. Maybe this means calling a friend, listening to music, walking the dog, or working out. Fill up these pages and add to them as you want. Use this space for your creative flow! You can doodle your ideas, or write them down. Take some time to reflect on this topic, and add to this list whenever something strikes you. Every day, pick one thing from this list that you will do to ensure you took an extra step toward your self-care for the day.

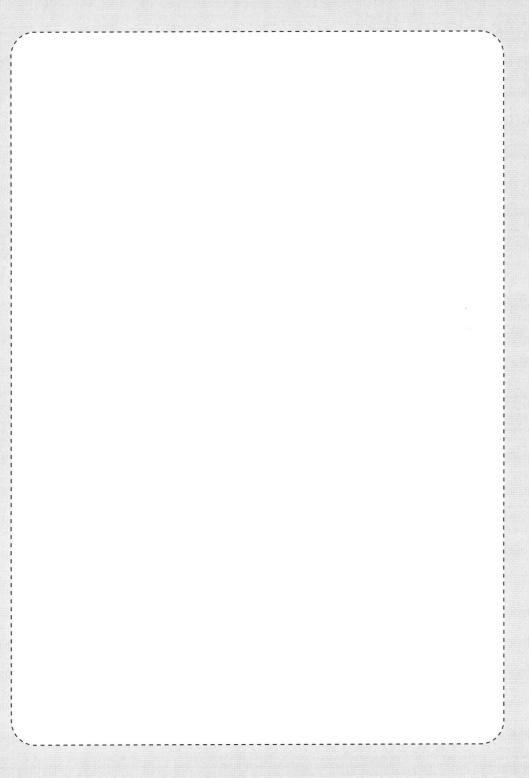

WEEKLY JOURNALING

To follow, you will find your first seven days of journaling. Begin your week of daily journaling now that you have concluded the above section and your "Joy & Meaning" pages. Once you have completed the seven days of journaling, read the next chapter. You will have a week of journaling after each weekly chapter, to allow you time to assimilate each week's content and homework assignments.

> **PRO TIP:** You can always start a deeper journaling practice by getting something as simple as a spiral bound note pad to record your thoughts in. Nothing fancy required!

Sometimes it is hard to get started writing in a journal. Here are some thoughtful questions for journaling inspiration:

- How was your day today?

- Where is your favorite place in the world? It could be your backyard, favorite beach or park, a friend's house, a town, your car, a room in your house or anywhere that speaks to you. Why is this place your "Happy Place?"

- If a crystal ball could tell you the truth about yourself, your life, the future, or anything else, what would you want to know?

- What is the greatest accomplishment of your life?

- What do you value most in a friendship?

- What is your favorite memory? Why?

- Who inspires you? Why are they an inspiration?

- What makes you unique?

- What is the best compliment you ever received?

- If you had a theme song, what would it be?

- What is your favorite song? Is there a memory or feeling attached to that song? Why do you like that song?

- What is a habit you would like to change?

- What couldn't you live without?

- What makes you feel content?

- What do you wish others knew about you?

- What is the best advice someone ever gave you? Why?

- What do you want to be remembered for?

- What friends are you most grateful for? List what makes each friend so special.

- If my body could talk, what would it say to me?

- What is your favorite piece of clothing? Why is it so special to you?

- What would you like to learn, do or try in your life? Write these things down and start checking them off as you complete them.

Day 1: YOUR HEART TO SOUL DAILY JOURNAL

DATE: _____

DAILY WEIGHT:_____ A.M. GLUCOSE:_____

TODAY'S OVERALL FEELING OF WELLNESS:

1   2   3   4   5   6   7   8   9   10

INTENTION WORD FOR THE DAY:_____

TODAY I ACCOMPLISHED:

☐ Mindful breath work

☐ Mindful meditation (Duration _____)

☐ Joy & Meaning self-care activity:_____

3 THINGS I AM GRATEFUL FOR TODAY:

1.

2.

3.

WHAT'S ON YOUR MIND?

Day 2: **YOUR HEART TO SOUL DAILY JOURNAL**

DATE: _____

DAILY WEIGHT:_____ A.M. GLUCOSE:_____

TODAY'S OVERALL FEELING OF WELLNESS:

1   2   3   4   5   6   7   8   9   10

INTENTION WORD FOR THE DAY:_____

TODAY I ACCOMPLISHED:

☐ Mindful breath work

☐ Mindful meditation (Duration _____)

☐ Joy & Meaning self-care activity:_____

3 THINGS I AM GRATEFUL FOR TODAY:

1.

2.

3.

WHAT'S ON YOUR MIND?

Day 3: YOUR HEART TO SOUL DAILY JOURNAL

DATE: _____

DAILY WEIGHT:_____ A.M. GLUCOSE:_____

TODAY'S OVERALL FEELING OF WELLNESS:

1   2   3   4   5   6   7   8   9   10

INTENTION WORD FOR THE DAY:_____

TODAY I ACCOMPLISHED:

☐ Mindful breath work

☐ Mindful meditation (Duration _____)

☐ Joy & Meaning self-care activity:_____

3 THINGS I AM GRATEFUL FOR TODAY:

1.

2.

3.

WHAT'S ON YOUR MIND?

Day 4: YOUR HEART TO SOUL DAILY JOURNAL

DATE: _____

DAILY WEIGHT: _____   A.M. GLUCOSE: _____

TODAY'S OVERALL FEELING OF WELLNESS:

1   2   3   4   5   6   7   8   9   10

INTENTION WORD FOR THE DAY: _____

TODAY I ACCOMPLISHED:

- ☐ Mindful breath work
- ☐ Mindful meditation (Duration _____)
- ☐ Joy & Meaning self-care activity: _____

3 THINGS I AM GRATEFUL FOR TODAY:

1.

2.

3.

WHAT'S ON YOUR MIND?

Day 5: YOUR HEART TO SOUL DAILY JOURNAL

DATE: _____

DAILY WEIGHT: _____ A.M. GLUCOSE: _____

TODAY'S OVERALL FEELING OF WELLNESS:

1   2   3   4   5   6   7   8   9   10

INTENTION WORD FOR THE DAY: _____

TODAY I ACCOMPLISHED:

☐ Mindful breath work

☐ Mindful meditation (Duration _____)

☐ Joy & Meaning self-care activity: _____

3 THINGS I AM GRATEFUL FOR TODAY:

1.

2.

3.

WHAT'S ON YOUR MIND?

Day 6: YOUR HEART TO SOUL DAILY JOURNAL

DATE: _____

DAILY WEIGHT: _____ A.M. GLUCOSE: _____

TODAY'S OVERALL FEELING OF WELLNESS:

1   2   3   4   5   6   7   8   9   10

INTENTION WORD FOR THE DAY: _____

TODAY I ACCOMPLISHED:

☐ Mindful breath work

☐ Mindful meditation (Duration _____)

☐ Joy & Meaning self-care activity: _____

3 THINGS I AM GRATEFUL FOR TODAY:

1.

2.

3.

WHAT'S ON YOUR MIND?

Day 7: YOUR HEART TO SOUL DAILY JOURNAL

DATE: _____

DAILY WEIGHT: _____ A.M. GLUCOSE: _____

TODAY'S OVERALL FEELING OF WELLNESS:

1   2   3   4   5   6   7   8   9   10

INTENTION WORD FOR THE DAY: _____

TODAY I ACCOMPLISHED:

☐ Mindful breath work

☐ Mindful meditation (Duration _____)

☐ Joy & Meaning self-care activity: _____

3 THINGS I AM GRATEFUL FOR TODAY:

1.

2.

3.

WHAT'S ON YOUR MIND?

Week 2:
TURN SURVIVAL INTO "THRIVAL"

How are we doing so far? Take a moment to check-in with yourself and observe all the changes you have already made in only one week!

As part of your self-care, you can use your food as your "Nutritional Farm-acy" to decrease the need of having to go to an actual pharmacy for medication. Nutrition from foods can help heal you by *preventing* inflammation and disease. Everything we put on the end of our fork moves our body to either a state of wellness or to a state of inflammation and illness.

Food can be your "culinary medicine," your healing preventive medicine against diseases. Imagine if you tried to grow an apple tree and instead of soil you planted it in potato chips and hamburgers and watered it with soda, and you kept it inside all day out of the sun, in front of a TV. How would that apple tree grow? Can you grow a living tree, or your living body, by feeding it dead food products? Lifestyle choices like what you feed your body, how often you exercise and get sun and fresh air outdoors, all matter. Like the apple tree, your body cannot thrive when fed dead "food products."

INFLAMMATION

Let's talk about inflammation, which is key to understanding how food can work for you or against you, and why. Inflammation is your body's natural response against things that threaten it, including infections, injuries, and toxins, so that it can rebalance itself. When your body detects a threat, it releases chemicals that trigger a response from your immune system, which tries to repair it. The tricky part is this: you may be unaware that your body is suffering from inflammation. You may not have glaring symptoms, until over time, your body manifests an illness.

This inflammatory fight response includes the release of antibodies and proteins, as well as increased blood flow to the damaged area. The whole process usually lasts a few hours, or days in the case of acute (recent onset) inflammation.

Chronic (long term/ongoing) inflammation happens when this inflammatory response lingers, leaving your body in a constant state of alertness. Over time, chronic inflammation may have a negative impact on your tissues and organs.

Inflammation may inhibit the release of nitric oxide, a chemical your body releases that opens your blood vessels. If your blood vessels are not dilated, it makes your heart work harder and can put you at risk for clots, strokes, and heart attacks.

A major factor contributing to inflammation is the consumption of animal products including milk, all dairy and all meats, eggs, fatty foods, fried foods, excess alcohol, oils, processed foods, sodas, and sugary drinks and for some people, foods containing gluten, (found in wheat, spelt, kamut, farro, durum, bulgur, semolina, barley, rye, tricale and gluten containing oats). What? This sounds like all foods, right? I know, I felt that way, too at the beginning of my own wellness journey. Let's take a closer look here at what is going on. Don't worry—we are still going to have fun with food. Calm down, taste buds!

Environmental toxins in and on our food, such as pesticides and airborne toxins, can cause inflammation in our bodies. Is your food full of pesticides, herbicides, chemicals, food additives, food preservatives, food dyes, genetically altered food, polluted crops from air pollution and chem trails? It's often hard or impossible to answer this question, until you become a detective in your own eating habits and investigate where your food comes from.

Reflection Questions: We must consider the *sourcing* of our food. What is on the end of your fork and *how did it get there*? Where did it come from? How was it grown and what was added to it? Was it made in a factory? What are the ingredients? What does your plate look like when you are done eating? Is it full of grease or oil? How is the quality of the water you drink? Have you considered testing your drinking water for possible contaminants?

> PRO TIP: There are water test kits you can order, and some water pitcher filters come with a test so you can see when it is time to change the filter.

WHAT CAN WE DO TO PROTECT OURSELVES FROM INFLAMMATION? HERE IS A SIMPLE GUIDELINE:

If your food was *made* in a processing plant, you may want to avoid it, or not have it much. But if it come from the ground and if it *is a fresh plant* (fruit or vegetable) from the grocery store, garden or farmer's market, enjoy it. To quote Michael Pollan, the author of *The Omnivore's Dilemma: A Natural History of Four Meals*, when asked about the healthiest way to eat: "Eat food. Not too much. Mostly plants."

First, cut back on the following foods, below. Remember that these changes outlined throughout the book don't have to be all at once and overnight. Don't be frightened. As with everything else in this heart and wellness journey, it all starts with small changes. A change becomes a habit, and a habit becomes a lifestyle. Taking little steps is progress forward, and continuing to move forward to your health goals is the key.

The (ultimate) goal is to cut back on **all** animal products from your body, all forms of dairy, including milk and cheese, all meats, even chicken and fish and eggs. Eliminate fatty foods. Minimize using oils in meal preparation. Steer clear of the call of fried foods, foods containing gluten, excess alcohol, processed foods, sodas and sugary drinks. Go gluten-free as much as possible. Certain foods containing gluten may cause inflammation for some people. Don't worry! We will learn how to step into this gradually.

Why do we want to cut down on these foods? These inflammatory foods create an acidic environment in your body where cancer and inflammation have been known to thrive. Some studies have shown that acidic environments may help cancer cells grow. A diet low in these acidic foods can help the body to raise its pH level, (the acid/base balance in the body chemistry) thus acting as a deterrent for the growth of cancer cells. Have you heard of someone curing their cancer by eating bacon? No, because bacon, an acidifying, inflammatory, fatty food, has been proven to cause cancer. Fruits and vegetables help the body become more alkaline and empower our body to be able to bring us back to wellness. The story of Kris Carr, author of *Crazy Sexy Cancer Survivor* is very inspiring. Kris has managed to halt the growth and spread of inoperable cancers in herself by following a plant-based lifestyle. Kris is simply too sexy for her cancer now, and you, likewise can be too cool for heart disease! Let's get your arteries to act like they are coated with Teflon, so your blood can flow easily and your heart keeps on doing its work with ease. How do we begin?

EAT ANTIOXIDANTS

Inflammatory toxins produce rogue unstable molecules called free radicals. Free radicals cause oxidation inside our body, kind of like the brown rust you would find on an old metal fence. These free radical mischief makers try to take an electron (molecular energy transmitter) from any possible source. Antioxidants kindly volunteer themselves to give up an electron to neutralize the free radical, preventing damage to the body. Antioxidants, found in the rainbow of vibrant colors of fresh fruits and vegetables, are our superhero inflammation fighters. By eating a wide selection of colorful fruits and vegetables we can get a variety of antioxidants and nutrients.

As much as possible, eat locally raised fresh organic produce, to support your local farmer's markets. Buying produce from local farmers helps your local economy, avoids the cost of fuel and prevents environmental harm to air quality from shipping the produce. Buy produce more frequently to get the freshest produce and to avoid wasting perishable food. Buying organic food and purchasing your produce at farmer's markets may seem expensive, but is well worth it. Fruits and vegetables, rice and beans and vegan meals cost less than meat, prescription medications, doctor visits and missed work. The money spent on organic and healthy foods is an *investment* in your health. Let your food become your "Farm-acy," as renowned functional medicine physician Dr. Mark Hyman says.

> **Hospital bills, doctor's visits, medical tests, time off from missed work, emotional duress, the cost of transportation to and from medical appointments, and expensive medications waste our money, time, and energy.**

FOOD DESERTS

It is not always easy or affordable for everyone to have access to healthy food. Across the country there are areas called "food deserts," meaning that there are urban and rural areas across the country that only offer fast food or pre-packaged food in convenience stores. Per Kelly Brooks, author of the spring 2014 issue of Johns Hopkins magazine article "Research Shows Food Deserts More Abundant in Minority Neighborhoods," "Food deserts are found in low-income, predominantly Black and Hispanic communities. Because of their lack of healthy food, people living in food deserts are associated with having a higher incidence of cardiac disease, obesity, and diabetes. Obesity and diabetes increase inflammation in the body, triggering further illness like heart disease."

Plant-based critical care physician and member of The Physicians Committee for Responsible Medicine, (PCRM), Dr. Milton Mills states: "Animal protein and animal fat causes elevated levels of inflammation, which dampens down immune function and they also directly interfere with the ability of the immune cells to do their job." Dr. Mills says further: "Studies have shown that people living under systemic and society wide racism and are encountering specific racially motivated actions actually have stress genes that are turned on that promote inflammation and make them more susceptible to illness."

We can see how life in these food deserts can easily lead to obesity, increased inflammation, diabetes, heart disease and increased illness. I saw this firsthand in many of my patients, when asking them what their eating habits were. I remember one patient telling me he thought that fried chicken, fries and a strawberry milkshake was a healthy meal because it contained meat (protein) dairy (calcium and protein) fruit (the strawberry flavoring) and a vegetable (fried potatoes). This deep-fried, saturated fat and sugar-laden meal of artificial colors and chemical lab-made flavors was an inferno of artery clogging inflammatory fats. Eating these foods is what led to this man having a massive heart attack. This was only one meal of his day, living in a food desert. Breakfast may have been a bacon egg and cheese sandwich, and for dinner; a burger, fries, and a soda from another fast food restaurant. We can clearly see how and why obesity, diabetes, and heart disease are rampant in people who live in these food deserts.

Consider the amount of time it takes to travel to doctor's visits, medical tests and to the pharmacy, and imagine that instead, you were to allocate this time toward visiting a market that has fresh fruits and vegetables. How could you do this if you live in a food desert? Could you rotate shopping with a group of people, maybe alternating, making a once-a-week trip? Would it be possible to shop in an off-hour time when it might be easier to take a bus or subway to the grocery store? Could you start your own food co-op in which you all pooled food? Are there food programs such as SNAP that you can enroll in? Is there a community garden that you could become a part of? Is there a lot or yard where you could create a garden? Could you get a neighbor involved in helping you by allowing you space to make a garden on their property, in trade for their own fresh produce? Can you reach out to your local government representative to help with finding access to a community garden to grow or purchase fresh fruits and vegetables? Can you form a group with others to purchase and get deliveries from a CSA (Community Supported Agriculture) farm? A CSA allows you to make an arrangement to purchase fresh produce directly from a farm and if there are enough people subscribing, maybe the farm can drop off your produce in a mutually convenient area for pickup. Look up localharvest.org to see what farms are participating and to begin your own CSA.

Eating in a way that maximizes the freshest foods—fruits and vegetables, which have as little packaging as possible—is an important way to control the inflammation that can lead to heart disease and other health conditions.

> **PRO TIP**: If you cannot get fresh produce, frozen produce is very good to use as a substitute.

Reflection Questions: If you have to go to a "health food" store, what does that make the grocery store? If you see a "health" aisle at the supermarket, what does that make the rest of the store's products?

> **PRO TIP**: Purchase a grocery shopping cart or large tote bags to help you organize and carry your shopping goods. Reusable tote bags are better for the environment and will help you organize your shopping.

OTHER WAYS TO COMBAT INFLAMMATION

Do not smoke. Smoking not only causes cancer, it constricts blood vessels and impedes blood flow to the heart and the other vital organs.

Minimize your exposure to environmental air pollution.

Get a water filter for your drinking water. Change the filters as recommended. Test the water if you have a test kit with your filter, or see if you can obtain an independent test kit.

Avoid excess sun. We need about 15 minutes of sun exposure per day. Those folks who live in areas like the cooler northern and northeastern United States get less sun than those living in sunny climates like California and Florida. Less sun exposure means you may have a deficiency in vitamin D, so it is a good idea to check your vitamin D levels with your doctor. vitamin D is important in helping our immune systems stay in top shape. If you plan to be in the sun longer than 15 minutes a day, especially between 10:00 a.m. and 2:00 p.m., it is important to apply sunscreen to prevent sunburn.

Avoid excess radiation. Turn off your Wi-Fi router when possible. Consider using cabled earbuds instead of wireless headphones or cordless earbuds for your phone. Keep your cell phone off and in another room when you sleep. Put your phone on "airplane" mode as much as possible when it is on.

Switch to healthier cleaning products for your home. Search online to find out how you can make your own home cleaning products, which are inexpensive and effective.

Exercise daily. Move your body at least 20–30 minutes a day, even if you start by simply walking. See your doctor to obtain their approval before starting any exercise program.

Get adequate rest and at least 7.5 hours of sleep each night. Sleep is important to help our body restore itself, and in helping our immune system stay strong.

Hydrate. Drink at least (8) eight-ounce glasses of water every day. If you are on diuretic medications or fluid restrictions, please check with your doctor about the adequate amount of fluids you should be drinking each day.

Avoid excess alcohol. Alcohol can interfere with the liver and its ability to screen and clean our blood. Alcohol can also lead to processes that harden the arteries and increase blood pressure, both which make the heart work harder.

Avoid recreational drugs. Cocaine has been known to induce heart attacks.

Avoid excess caffeine. Caffeine consumed after 12:00 p.m. can interfere with your sleep cycle. Although caffeine is a liquid, it is not water! Caffeinated beverages are very dehydrating. When having a caffeinated beverage, have a glass of water to replenish your fluids.

Add ground flax seeds, ground chia seeds or chopped walnuts to your food for anti-inflammatory Omega 3 benefits.

Avoid sugary foods. This includes the hidden danger of high fructose corn syrup. This form of fructose is not used directly by our muscles for energy; instead, it goes to the liver, which in response brings up triglyceride levels, which contributes to heart disease.

Manage your stress levels. Stress negatively affects our immune system by decreasing the ability of our white blood cells to fight infection. Stress also causes inflammation, which is why exercise (with your doctor's permission) meditation, self-care time, hobbies that calm you, and sharing time communicating with good friends and loving family are so important for stress reduction. Spend quality time with friends and family who you can share laughter and good times with. Practice breath work and meditation. Reference the section in Part Three of this book called "Pre-Op: Preparing For Your Heart Surgery." There are lots of recommendations there which will help you to reduce your stress and calm your mind.

Alleviate *localized* inflammation. Applying topical organic CBD (Cannabidiol, an active component of the hemp plant) salve or balm is wonderful for easing localized spot inflammation and pain. At this time, I recommend *topical use only* until more research and scientific data is available regarding the interactions of medications with CBD. Do not apply CBD salve or CBD products directly to an open wound. Introducing a product onto an open wound could cause an infection.

Now that we have addressed inflammation, which can lead to heart disease and other illnesses, let's optimize your immune system further, so your body will be an inhospitable host for disease.

HOMEOSTASIS

Homeostasis is the body's natural healthy state of balance. Despite what we do to it or put into it, our bodies are constantly trying to maintain this balanced state.

In addition to decreasing the inflammation in our bodies to promote homeostasis, what else can we do? We can create an environment in our body that is inhospitable for disease, bacteria, fungus, and viruses. Viruses, funguses and bacteria need a host—a human body. The host (you) serves as their residence. Eating inflammatory foods provides an environment so the body not only hosts, but also *welcomes* bacteria, fungus, viruses and their diseases. Let's roll up the welcome mat so they won't stop at our door anymore! How do we do that?

We optimize our health by decreasing inflammation and adding on antibacterial and antiviral foods, while supporting our gut bacteria so that bacteria, fungus and viruses will not have an environment to thrive in. *Treating every meal as wellness medicine* is so important because it makes it easier for our body to operate. We have over twenty-one opportunities a week (three meals a day times seven days, *plus* snacks) to make conscious choices about what we feed our body to help it optimize itself in homeostasis. Creating healthful homemade meals requires thoughtful shopping and time for preparation. Junk food is convenient and easy, but will bring you illnesses that were preventable and could lead to a possible early death.

Filmmaker Morgan Spurlock tested out if junk food could lead to illness in his movie *Super Size Me*, in which he ate nothing but fast food from a popular chain restaurant for thirty days. Spurlock gained weight, lost energy and motivation, and felt like he was headed for an early death. The takeaway from *Super Size Me* is that the "Standard American Diet" can lead to the "Standard American Diseases," which in turn lead to the "Standard American Medications!" I recall this phrase by the mnemonic:

SAD   SAD   SAM

Please note that by the "Standard American Medications," I am referring to medications that may not otherwise be needed if a person had been able to make other healthier lifestyle choices. Some of the same medications may also be used in saving someone else's life. It is not too late to improve your health and to avoid unnecessary medications that are a consequence of poor nutritional intake. Due to your personal health history, you may need certain medications. Always speak with your doctor about any concerns you have regarding your medications. Certain medications may be a necessity for your health condition, and this is why it is important for you to know and understand why you are taking each medication.

HOW CAN WE OPTIMIZE OURSELVES WITH OUR FOODS?

What can we do with food to help our bodies maintain homeostasis? A huge part of our health and wellness all comes back to what is on the end of your fork and what you put into your mouth.

Alkalize. Start your day with the juice from half a lemon mixed into a cup of room temperature water to alkalize the body. While you may think "But lemon is acidic!" Lemon is metabolized by the body and produces alkaline byproducts, making us a less hospitable host to disease.

Avoid cold or iced drinks, as they decrease the digestive fire. Your body is trying to heat up and metabolize digestion. Cold fluids are not helpful in this process, which requires incredible energy. Think about it: our body is taking what we put into our mouth, extracting what it can use, and eliminating what it doesn't want, all through one long connected system. That is really incredible, right?!

Eat and cook with antiviral and antibacterial herbs and foods. Cook with foods such as rosemary, thyme, sage, oregano, onion, garlic and leeks. Throw a pinch of herbs into your room temperature or warm glass of water or tea and let them infuse in it and flavor it. As the *Journal of Applied Microbiology*, Volume 95 / Issue 3, reports: "Many traditional plants have been reported to have strong antiviral activity and some of them have already been used to treat animals and people who suffer from viral infection." I encourage you to research more about the healing antiviral and antimicrobial properties of these simple common herbs in relation to bacteria and viruses. I love cooking with rosemary because it adds such a nice homey flavor. I use it in pasta, potato dishes, homemade hummus, and even chopped finely on a fresh fruit salad.

Cook with anti-inflammatory foods such as turmeric and ginger.
Turmeric must be cooked with black pepper in order for the body
to optimally absorb the turmeric to get its full benefits. Ginger is
known for its warming properties and as a digestive aid. Consider
how ginger ale is taken for an upset stomach.

Seed and Feed. Seed or populate your gut with probiotics, the "good"
bacteria residing in your gut, which form the basis of your immunity.
Probiotics are made of good live bacteria and/or yeasts that naturally live in your body. You can have both good and bad bacteria in
your body. When you get an infection, the bad bacteria take over,
increasing in number, which creates an imbalance. Populating your
gut by *adding* the good bacteria found in probiotics into your nutrition increases the number of good bacteria, which helps to eliminate
bad bacteria, restores gut balance, and allows your body to prevent
infection. Probiotic foods are a way to add good bacteria to your body
to fight the bad bacteria. Probiotics are found added in dairy-free
"yogurts," and in fermented foods such as miso, kombucha drinks,
tempeh, sauerkraut, sourdough bread, kimchi, and pickles.

Now that you have added good bacteria to your gut, feed them!
Your new good gut bacteria love prebiotic foods. Prebiotics are dietary
fibers that act like fertilizer to help feed the friendly, good bacteria
in your gut. Prebiotics are found in foods such as flax, nuts, seeds,
artichokes, leeks, garlic, onion, asparagus, seaweed, beans, potatoes,
bananas, apples, apricots, and oranges.

WEEKLY HOMEWORK
(CHECK OFF WHEN COMPLETED)

☐ Try out a "Meatless Monday!" Take all animal products out of Mondays to gradually make a move to healthier eating habits. Could you have oatmeal for breakfast instead of eggs and bacon? Could you try a veggie burger option for lunch instead of a beef burger? How might you feel after a dinner of salad and rice and beans with vegetables instead of chicken? Search online for your favorite meat dish and replace it with the word "vegan," (no animal meat in the food) as in "vegan pasta dishes." How creative can you get making a day of it? If you can make a day of it, can you make a week of it? Can you then make a lifestyle of it? Maybe new healthy family traditions become an offshoot of your positive lifestyle changes. One day, one meal at a time and you will be surprised by how tasty your food is and how much you stop craving meat, added sugars, and even fast food. I love the recipes in Robin Quivers' book: *The Vegucation of Robin*. She makes healing food preparation so easy (and tasty!)

☐ Experiment with eating a probiotic (examples: coconut non-dairy yogurt with live "good" bacterial cultures or a kombucha drink) and prebiotic (examples: bananas, garlic, asparagus and many more veggies and fruits) foods this week. Remember we want to first seed (add the probiotic) then feed it (with a prebiotic).

☐ Watch the movie *Super Size Me* (2004) available online.

☐ Explore new stores or farmer's markets where you can shop for healthier food. Grab a buddy to go with you on this journey.

Day 8: YOUR HEART TO SOUL DAILY JOURNAL

DATE: _____

DAILY WEIGHT: _____ A.M. GLUCOSE: _____

TODAY'S OVERALL FEELING OF WELLNESS:

1   2   3   4   5   6   7   8   9   10

INTENTION WORD FOR THE DAY: _____

TODAY I ACCOMPLISHED:

☐ Mindful breath work

☐ Mindful meditation (Duration _____)

☐ Joy & Meaning self-care activity: _____

3 THINGS I AM GRATEFUL FOR TODAY:

1.

2.

3.

WHAT'S ON YOUR MIND?

Day 9: YOUR HEART TO SOUL DAILY JOURNAL

DATE: _____

DAILY WEIGHT: _____ A.M. GLUCOSE: _____

TODAY'S OVERALL FEELING OF WELLNESS:

1   2   3   4   5   6   7   8   9   10

INTENTION WORD FOR THE DAY: _____

TODAY I ACCOMPLISHED:

☐ Mindful breath work

☐ Mindful meditation (Duration _____)

☐ Joy & Meaning self-care activity: _____

3 THINGS I AM GRATEFUL FOR TODAY:

1.

2.

3.

WHAT'S ON YOUR MIND?

Day 10: YOUR HEART TO SOUL DAILY JOURNAL

DATE: _____

DAILY WEIGHT: _____   **A.M. GLUCOSE:** _____

TODAY'S OVERALL FEELING OF WELLNESS:

1   2   3   4   5   6   7   8   9   10

INTENTION WORD FOR THE DAY: _____

TODAY I ACCOMPLISHED:

☐ Mindful breath work

☐ Mindful meditation (Duration _____)

☐ Joy & Meaning self-care activity: _____

3 THINGS I AM GRATEFUL FOR TODAY:

1.

2.

3.

WHAT'S ON YOUR MIND?

Day 11: YOUR HEART TO SOUL DAILY JOURNAL

DATE: _____

DAILY WEIGHT: _____   **A.M. GLUCOSE:** _____

TODAY'S OVERALL FEELING OF WELLNESS:

1   2   3   4   5   6   7   8   9   10

INTENTION WORD FOR THE DAY: _____

TODAY I ACCOMPLISHED:

☐ Mindful breath work

☐ Mindful meditation (Duration _____)

☐ Joy & Meaning self-care activity: _____

3 THINGS I AM GRATEFUL FOR TODAY:

1.

2.

3.

WHAT'S ON YOUR MIND?

Day 12: YOUR HEART TO SOUL DAILY JOURNAL

DATE: _____

DAILY WEIGHT: _____ A.M. GLUCOSE: _____

TODAY'S OVERALL FEELING OF WELLNESS:

1   2   3   4   5   6   7   8   9   10

INTENTION WORD FOR THE DAY: _____

TODAY I ACCOMPLISHED:

☐ Mindful breath work

☐ Mindful meditation (Duration _____)

☐ Joy & Meaning self-care activity: _____

3 THINGS I AM GRATEFUL FOR TODAY:

1.

2.

3.

WHAT'S ON YOUR MIND?

Day 13: YOUR HEART TO SOUL DAILY JOURNAL

DATE: _____

DAILY WEIGHT:_____   A.M. GLUCOSE:_____

TODAY'S OVERALL FEELING OF WELLNESS:

1   2   3   4   5   6   7   8   9   10

INTENTION WORD FOR THE DAY:_____

TODAY I ACCOMPLISHED:

☐ Mindful breath work

☐ Mindful meditation (Duration _____)

☐ Joy & Meaning self-care activity:_____

3 THINGS I AM GRATEFUL FOR TODAY:

1.

2.

3.

WHAT'S ON YOUR MIND?

Day 14: YOUR HEART TO SOUL DAILY JOURNAL

DATE: _____

DAILY WEIGHT:_____   A.M. GLUCOSE:_____

TODAY'S OVERALL FEELING OF WELLNESS:

1   2   3   4   5   6   7   8   9   10

INTENTION WORD FOR THE DAY:_____

TODAY I ACCOMPLISHED:

☐ Mindful breath work

☐ Mindful meditation (Duration _____)

☐ Joy & Meaning self-care activity:_____

3 THINGS I AM GRATEFUL FOR TODAY:

1.

2.

3.

WHAT'S ON YOUR MIND?

Week 3:

THE "CARDIAC BERMUDA TRIANGLE"

We are off to a great start, learning to nurture ourselves with self-care, and using breath work and meditation to help us become more relaxed. We have seen how we can use prebiotics and probiotics, and herbs and spices in our food to boost our health. We have learned how to protect ourselves from inflammation, a root cause of many diseases. Now let's get to some nuts and bolts behind how and why we get sick.

Let's take a look at how we unfortunately put a stamp on our body's passport, enabling us to travel to the "Cardiac Bermuda Triangle." (Please note: the "Cardiac Bermuda Triangle" is unrelated to the beautiful archipelago of Bermuda and its islands.)

The "Cardiac Bermuda Triangle" consists of the "highs" of cardiac disease: *high blood pressure*, *high cholesterol and fats* in the arteries and cells, and *high blood sugar* found in Type 2 diabetes.

HYPERTENSION (HIGH BLOOD PRESSURE)

Hold your fist up in front of you and open and close it while you are reading this paragraph. I will let you know when to stop pumping your fist. Your heart is approximately the same size as your fist. Now look at your fist in comparison to the rest of your body size. Your heart has to pump out an average of 5 liters of blood per minute. Consider what (5) one-liter bottles of soda look like. Your heart is pumping that blood through all that real estate of your body every minute. Is your fist still pumping? Keep going! We are not done with our paragraph yet. Your heart is literally pumping the equivalent of *swimming pools* worth of blood over the course of your lifetime. Your heart has to get your blood down to the tips of your toes and fingers and up to your head against gravity. Hypertension (high blood pressure), makes it harder for the heart to work to circulate the blood. Think of what happens if you kink a garden hose. That kink is increasing the pressure which is then backing up in the hose, and where does the pressure back up to? The spigot, or in this case, your heart. The same application of our hose pressure can be seen for your heart. If the arteries are clamped down and narrowed from hypertension, the blood has a tougher time pushing the blood through your system. Our arteries are like a freeway, with blood cells being the cars. If the freeway gets narrower, (hypertension) what happens to the cars? You have traffic, you have backups, you have accidents like blood clots and a heart attack. We don't want accidents! We want our blood to flow freely and our heart to be easy in its contractions. We need to make it easier on our heart to get blood through all of our body's real estate. You can stop clenching your fist now. That little exercise was to show you that your heart is in your chest doing a pushup on itself every second. Imagine, if your hand got a little tired there, how the heart is doing this non-stop pushup 100,000 times a day for 80 years or so. Let's take a moment to reflect on our new best friend, the heart.

HYPERLIPIDEMIA
(HIGH CHOLESTEROL AND TRIGLYCERIDES)

When we eat fatty foods, such as meats or deep-fried foods, and all those things that may taste good due to their saturated fat content, such as BBQ meats, bacon, fries, and donuts, they clog up our arteries so the blood cells (the cars in artery traffic) cannot get through. When we eat these foods, we are increasing the fat, cholesterol, and triglycerides (waxy, fat-like substances) in our blood. Would you pour bacon fat down your sink drain? You wouldn't because what would happen if you did? You would have a coating that would eventually block up your sink drain and pipes over time. This is exactly what happens when you eat any of these foods; over time, they block up your "pipes," the arteries. The lanes of your freeway are blocked off, and what is happening to the ability of the blood cells to move through your body to deliver oxygen and nutrients? They cannot work properly. What happens if you have hypertension AND you eat a lot of fatty foods? Right—you have blocked off your arteries, and have made it more difficult for the heart to pump effectively. Over time, we can have heart damage, valve failure, heart failure, a heart attack, a stroke, peripheral artery disease, arrhythmias, atherosclerosis, and more.

The "Cardiac Bermuda Triangle" can also lead to erectile dysfunction, a leading indicator that a man may have cardiac disease.

Clogged arteries are everywhere, including the vessels that bring blood to the penis. **Before you seek a prescription for erectile dysfunction medications, it is very important to see a cardiologist. If you are already taking an erectile enhancing medication, do let your doctor know.** Erectile enhancement medications act as a vasodilator, opening vessels to allow more blood to flow, which causes a drop in blood pressure. If a cardiologist did not know you were on these vasodilating medications and prescribed a medication which *also* acts as a vasodilator, and decreases your blood pressure, you could have a serious or possibly fatal drop in blood pressure. We will talk more about heart disease and the possibility for reversing it as we go along on our journey. Maybe by the end of our nine weeks together here, you can even look forward to *enhanced* erectile function. Talk about a powerful incentive!

TYPE 2 DIABETES (HIGH BLOOD SUGAR)

You may not have diabetes now or *yet*. Please continue reading this section because you will find out how diabetes manifests in our body, and how you can protect yourself from getting it.

"A NIGHT AT THE CLUB"

What happens in your body with Type 2 diabetes, and how you could get it over time. Let's imagine that a cell in your body is the coolest nightclub in town. In the nucleus (the center of the cell), there is a super exciting DJ playing your favorite music. The DJ has all the parts of the cell rocking out under a mirror ball and spotlights. The whole cell is twinkling, but it needs some more energy (which is created from glucose—our blood sugar) to keep the party going. Everybody wants to get into the club. Mr. Insulin (insulin is a blood-glucose controlling hormone made by a body organ called the pancreas) is a regular at the cell club with his girlfriend, Ms. Glucose. They always go on dates there at the cell. Mr. Insulin is a super cool guy, sharply dressed, with slicked back hair, and he is always wearing cool shoes. Ms. Glucose looks like a very edgy punk rocker with her spiky hairstyle. When Ms. Glucose enters the club, the party starts! Ms. Glucose cannot get into the club, though, unless she is escorted by Mr. Insulin. Mr. Insulin has his own VIP access to the club, and once he is in, he can let her into the club with her own access door. They each have special channels to enter through in the cell membrane. When we have Type 2 diabetes, insulin and glucose cannot get into the club. Why? Because there is a new bouncer in the club (the cell), and his name is "Fat." Fat is a big bouncer. He stands there at the entrance to the club with his arms crossed and he won't let insulin and glucose into the (cell) club. The fat from the foods you eat gets into your cells and doesn't allow insulin to escort glucose into cells for energy, so Type 2 diabetes—high blood sugar—is the result. Cells aren't able to receive the glucose energy they need to perform necessary functions in the body.

What does Ms. Glucose do if she can't get into the club? Ms. Glucose leaves the area in a huff to gather up with her glucose girlfriends, and because they all have spiky hairdos, and are wearing high heels, they wreak havoc, creating rips and tears on the artery walls, causing inflammation, which can enable plaque (fat and cholesterol) to build up there. Our bodies are smart, so they send our first responders (platelets—the kind of cells that form a scab outside the body) to stop a bleed that occurs if the artery is torn or plaque breaks off. The platelets come in with lights and sirens blaring to urgently patch the artery wall. The platelets work furiously, and the clot they make gets bigger until it blocks the artery off. Now there is no blood coming through. Uh oh! The body is now set up to have a heart attack.

A heart attack is lack of blood supply to the heart. Blood carries oxygen, and when the heart does not get oxygen it suffocates. Chest pain is the heart's gasps for oxygen. When the heart is hurt, it cries; it emits a protein called Troponin, which we can see from a blood test. If the artery is not opened in a timely manner, there can be huge damage to the heart muscle and its ability to pump. We can tell from an electrocardiogram (EKG) which artery is blocked and what part of the heart is damaged. We have gifted interventional cardiologists who are highly trained to get us out of this situation as quickly as possible by placing tubes called stents inside the area where the artery is blocked, to open the area up to restore blood flow. If there is too much blockage, heart surgeons have to bypass that area entirely, and this is called Coronary Artery Bypass Grafting, or CABG, an open-heart surgery where a vein from the leg or another area is grafted onto the blocked coronary artery to go around the blockage. Sometimes multiple coronary arteries have to be bypassed via surgery due to the blockages that have accrued over time from all these bad foods or other causes.

What happens to the artery freeways when we add Type 2 diabetes? The freeway is narrowed from hypertension, it is blocked off due to cholesterol and fats, and now with diabetes, the cars are driving in stickiness as if a truck full of pancake syrup spilled all over the freeway. A four-lane highway has become a slow, single file road for the (blood cell) cars. This now makes it even harder for the heart to pump. This is what happens when you take a trip to the "Cardiac Bermuda Triangle!"

TYPE 2 DIABETES

According to the American Diabetes Association, in 2018, 34.2 million Americans, or 10.5% of the population, had diabetes. Of the 34.2 million adults with diabetes, 26.8 million were diagnosed, and 7.4 million were undiagnosed.

In 2018, 10% of Americans had diabetes. That is 1 in 10 people. Many cases are still undiagnosed, so there are even more people with diabetes but they don't know they have it. This is why it is important to get your blood checked for diabetes.

Diabetes is rampant in our society, and yet it is silent. Like heart disease, you cannot see it. You may have diabetes, or pre-diabetes and not know it. It is important to see your doctor for tests, especially an A1c blood test, if you have any of the following signs and symptoms or risk factors for Type 2 diabetes:

- Feeling more tired than usual
- Urinating more than usual
- Extreme thirst
- Blurry vision
- Feeling hungrier than usual

- Losing weight without trying
- Dry, itchy skin
- Numbness and tingling in hands or feet

RISK FACTORS FOR TYPE 2 DIABETES:

- Overweight (recall your body mass index score that we recorded at the beginning of our 66 days?)
- 45 years or older
- Family member with Type 1 (the pancreas doesn't make insulin)
- Family member with Type 2
- Race/Ethnicity: Increased risk for people of color
- Smoking
- High blood pressure

Diabetes can cause numbness and tingling in the hands and feet and can lead to blindness, kidney failure, infections, and amputations of extremities. Diabetes negatively affects every organ of the body.

By taking the steps in this book, you not only will improve your heart health, you will be helping your body to avoid other diseases like diabetes as well.

I cared for hundreds of diabetic people during my 13-year nursing career in the cardiac ICU, and I always felt bad because these diabetic patients had to get their fingers pricked before each meal for a blood drop sample to measure their blood glucose level, then they had a shot of insulin immediately before each meal and possibly another shot of insulin before bedtime for overnight insulin coverage. The bouncer in their club was working overtime. These patients had up to seven needle pricks a day. Most all of our patients also got three injections of a blood thinning medication daily as a preventive measure against forming blood clots they could get from bedrest. For a severe diabetic, this treatment plan constituted up to ten or sometimes even more needle sticks a day.

In the hospital, especially after an operation, it is routine to closely monitor glucose levels and have tight glucose control achieved with insulin administration, even if you are not diabetic. Why are we so interested in keeping the sugar levels in our blood down, especially after open-heart surgery? Well, what loves sugar? Bacteria. And what do bacteria cause? Infection. We do not want infection after *any* surgery or procedure! Diabetics are more prone to infections for this reason. Let's work on stomping out diabetes while we are working on stomping out heart disease.

Now, let's add in smoking to see how it impacts the "Cardiac Bermuda Triangle." When you smoke, the arteries are constricted (narrowed) further. Why? Our bodies are so smart; they constrict the arteries to protect us from the entrance of this foreign smoke substance into the body. The problem is that there is also less oxygen to begin with because it is mixed with smoke, and now we have restricted the ability of oxygen to get to the cells and for the cells to move.

We are setting ourselves up for a heart attack again. We have narrowed the arteries from hypertension, narrowed them further with smoking, allowed in less oxygen, added grease so the artery walls are even narrower, and added sticky sugar that damaged the artery wall.

Are you beginning to see why cardiac disease has been the number one cause of death in the United States? How can we prevent the "Cardiac Bermuda Triangle" from happening?

ALL OF THESE SCENARIOS ARE POTENTIALLY REVERSIBLE!

How? First, stop smoking. Next, check what you have on the end of your fork. After that, adjust your rear view mirror and look at what's back there. That was where you and your old habits were. Now you are going to concentrate on your view out of the front windshield, and what lies ahead of you on your new road to wellness.

It all comes down to choices, and from those choices come consequences. According to the World Health Organization, processed meats have been scientifically shown, like cigarettes, to cause cancer.

Ultimately it could come down to that pepperoni and mozzarella pizza every Wednesday night or open-heart surgery, or diabetes, or cancer... Is it worth it?

> **What is the *risk* versus the *reward* in your food choices?**
>
> **(Taste buds are not allowed to answer this question!)**

Have you ever heard anyone tell you that they cured their cancer, asthma, obesity, diabetes or heart disease by eating more meat, cheese, dairy, donuts, burgers, and fries while taking fistfuls of medications to combat the illnesses rendered from those choices? Might this person be "playing themself?" So how do we fix our artery freeways so the blood cell cars can get around with ease, and the heart doesn't have additional stressors? How can we optimize our overall health? How can we get Ms. Glucose back in the club (the cell)? How can we get rid of Fat, the bouncer? If I told you that there was one thing you could do to change all of these things, even reverse them in your body, would you do it? Well, that's why we are here; to do just that!

> **The answer goes back to what is on your fork;**
> **is it healthy, or not?**

One of the first things I remember my nursing school professor, Ms. Norma Katz, telling us was, "Genetics loads the gun, but environment pulls the trigger." This means that while we have a certain genetic disposition that we are born with, what we do to our bodies can affect those genetics, and science has found that we can turn genes on and off by what we expose them to. Let's look at the following hypothetical story about identical twins, who had the same DNA, but their lifestyle choices led to different health outcomes.

These twins had identical genetic composition. Twin A lived in a smoggy city in a small apartment right by a noisy freeway. She routinely ate burgers and chips and soda and the only relation she had with any vegetable was that she was a couch potato. She had a callous on her right pointer finger from pushing the TV remote control button so much to change her TV channels. She was about 30 pounds overweight. She also smoked and loved drinking beer or whiskey each night. She was not a happy person and hated her job. She did not have many friends. She was depressed.

Twin B lived in a pretty and quiet suburb with lots of trees. She had nice neighbors, whom she considered her friends. Each morning she got up, meditated and went for a little jog before heading out to a job she enjoyed. She was a vegan because she did not believe in eating animals, and she felt that meat wasn't healthy for her body. She didn't like how her body felt after she ate meat. She had a dog and a cat she loved, and they brought her great joy. She did not smoke. She had a glass of red wine with dinner when she went out with friends on occasion. She loved tending her garden, reading mystery novels, and watching history shows when she did watch TV. She was upbeat and happy.

Which twin do you think is most likely to have cardiac disease, diabetes or cancer? Their genetics were the same; it was their *environment and lifestyles* which can trigger positive and negative gene expression, causing both negative and positive health conditions to manifest.

> **Disease prevention is so important.**
>
> **It is easier to *stay* healthy than to *get* healthy.**

If you had a car, and you drove with the parking brake on, never filled the radiator with water, never had the oil or oil filter changed, had no tread on the tires, the tires were low on air, over time, how would that car operate? You can find the best mechanics in town to "fix" your car each time it needs servicing, but that car will eventually break down again and again. Consider the owner of a car who has it routinely maintained, fills it with the best gas, drives it with ease, washes and shines it, inside and out, and takes it in for regular tune-ups and servicing. Might that car run better?

This is what happens to our bodies if we don't maintain them well. We have to go to see doctors (the "mechanics") to fix problems. If we are taking care of our body, tuning it up with the "mechanic" (our doctor) checking it routinely, preventing disease, aiding it in homeostasis, we are less likely to need a doctor to become a costly "mechanic."

"THE BEST DOCTOR IS NOT AN AUTHORITY FIGURE WHO WRITES PRESCRIPTIONS, BUT RATHER A PARTNER IN HEALING-SOMEONE WHO SEES PATIENTS IN THEIR FULLEST HUMANITY AND EMPOWERS THEM TO TAKE CHARGE OF THEIR HEALTH."

—DR. VIVEK MURTHY, nineteenth Surgeon General of the United States

----

It is very important that we see a doctor annually for a routine check-up, and when health concerns arise, however, the responsibility for your health and disease *prevention* is *your* responsibility and within *your own power.* You are in the driver's seat now. You are not the passenger anymore. YOU are the guardian of your health.

> **The negative experience of disease can be viewed as a positive catalyst to evaluate your lifestyle, activating you to make positive, course-corrective changes that will improve your health.**

The following story is about my first day as a nurse, and my first patient ever, "Zack." (Zack was not the patient's real name, nor was this the patient's age, to protect patient information and confidentiality.) Zack got another chance to make changes in his lifestyle which would prevent him from getting sicker. Most of the illnesses we have been talking about so far are the result of choices in lifestyle. Zack's story is a perfect example of illness caused by lifestyle choices.

As a fresh grad out of nursing school, I worked in the elite CCU- the Cardiac Care Unit, also known as the Cardiac ICU, the crown jewel in the tiara of the New York City public hospitals, at the oldest public hospital in the United States, serving the sickest of the sick. The pressure was on.

Our cardiac care unit was special because we did procedures that required the complexity, intervention, and care that other city public hospitals did not have the equipment or highly trained healthcare professionals to provide.

As a newly hired nurse, I was paired up with my trainer, Ted, (not his real name) who had been a former military nurse. Ted did not play. I was now "enlisted" in "Ted's Boot Camp." His work schedule was my work schedule. When he barked at me to do something, it had to happen, and it had to be executed perfectly and sooner rather than later. Ted did not want to ask for something twice. In fact, Ted wanted you to *anticipate* what was needed so that he didn't even have to ask you to do it. I wondered… "What kind of mind game is nursing?!" Having to ask for something made Ted impatient. Ted worked with a lot of new nurses like me and we all wanted to have Ted feel "at ease." Ted may not have been patient at times, but he was a fantastic teacher for me. Anticipating what is needed while keeping in mind preparations for alternative possible outcomes is key to being a top-notch nurse.

Ted and I listened to the 7:00 a.m. report from the outgoing night nurse. She had left us in good shape with our patient, acting fast upon his arrival which had only been a few minutes before. She told us that our patient, a 42-year-old male named Zack, had just been admitted to the cardiac ICU. Zack had a family history of cardiac disease. Both of his parents had suffered heart attacks. Zack had a personal history of hypertension, high cholesterol, and he was a smoker and overweight. (Do you notice any key parts of the "Cardiac Bermuda Triangle" in Zack's health history?) Zack was a member of a motorcycle club. I noticed his weathered, black leather motorcycle club jacket hanging from the bedside chair, the bright red bandana that he wore under his helmet cascading out of the front left pocket.

Zack had been out with other members of his motorcycle club the night before, where he had enjoyed many beers, deep fried Buffalo wings, a big steak dinner with fries, and ice cream for dessert. Zack had a few cigarettes and jokes with his buddies and then had ridden his motorcycle to his girlfriend's house. In the early morning he started to have chest pain. When the pain became "like an elephant sitting on his chest," he told his girlfriend to call 9-1-1.

As the outgoing night nurse was giving her report, we were simultaneously assessing Zack, feeling his pulse, listening to his heart and lungs and assessing him briefly, head to toe. Zack was sitting up in bed, and the monitor reflected his blood pressure was still a little high after two nitroglycerine tablets. His heart rate was variable. He was on a nasal cannula providing him with oxygen, yet he still appeared short of breath and was perspiring. He stated his pain had gone from a 10/10 to an 8/10 after the medication. Zack was hooked up to a portable defibrillator, and its heart rate tracing made a bleeping sound with each beat. An aide was getting a stretcher ready to transport Zack, the pack of emergency medications and syringes tucked under the head of the stretcher.

From their brief assessment and EKG upon Zack's arrival, the cardiology team determined Zack was having a "STEMI," a severe heart attack. We had to transport Zack upstairs to the Catheterization (Cath) Lab immediately, where they could assess and possibly fix any blockages to his coronary arteries. The Cath Lab team was ready for Zack and the room was prepared. "Let's go!" Ted commanded. "Time is muscle!" The longer Zack was delayed from getting to the procedure, the more heart muscle damage could occur. We grabbed the stretcher and called out to a doctor to join us for transport to the Cath Lab as we passed the cardiology team call room. The four of us were on the move.

It was only five minutes into my first nursing shift.

Two hours later, Ted and I got a call from the Cath Lab. They wanted to give us their report about the procedure and inform us that Zack was ready to be picked up and returned to his room on our unit.

Cath Lab reported that Zack had to have stents (medical devices shaped like supportive tubes) placed in two of his main coronary arteries to unblock them. Ironically, one of the blocked arteries was nicknamed in the medical industry as "The Widowmaker" and Zack's wife was now waiting in his hospital room. Zack's girlfriend was in the waiting room. Neither one knew of the other, but Zack sure knew them both!

Upon hearing this dilemma, Zack started to become upset and his heart rate became irregular on the monitor. We asked him what he wanted us to do to help him out with this situation.

We met his girlfriend a few minutes later when we returned Zack to his room. We had to jockey a few things around, but that is for another book.

Zack's story is a good one. He had the chance to make a turn-around in his health. Zack vowed that he was going to make changes to his lifestyle, starting from that day forward. He knew that he had been making poor choices and doing bad things to his body by smoking, eating poorly, and drinking in excess, which wasn't fair to himself or to those he cared about.

WHAT YOU AREN'T CHANGING, YOU ARE CHOOSING

In closing this chapter, I want to call up what I personally term "High Cardiac Season." December seemed to always be the month when we had the most patients. The Cardiac CCU was running non-stop with extra patients boarded in other ICUs because we ran out of rooms in the cardiac unit, and I always wondered why we had so many more patients then. In reflecting back through the years, this was my personal observation: December is a holiday time when people overeat, and travel on planes making them at risk for blood clots (remember how a blood clot can contribute to a heart attack). In December, people consume rich, heavy, fatty holiday meals, go to lots of parties, drink too much alcohol, may experiment with or do drugs, and have family drama with emotional stressors. December is also when shoveling snow may be necessary, when a person is not used to this physical exertion. All of these factors can contribute to "High Cardiac Season."

> **How might you be able to avoid "High Cardiac Season?"**

WEEKLY HOMEWORK
(CHECK OFF WHEN COMPLETED)

- ☐ Reflect for a moment about everything you ate yesterday, and so far today. What did you eat? Why did you eat it? When did you eat it? Why did you make that particular food choice? Were these healthy choices that nourished your body?

- ☐ Watch any online episode of Anthony Bourdain's *Parts Unknown*. Reflect on how we learn to culturally assimilate our possibly unhealthy foods.

- ☐ Listen to the Rich Roll Podcast episode 499 for stories and excellent information from the authors below on Type 1 and 2 diabetes.

- ☐ **If you are diabetic**, pick up a copy of the book *Mastering Diabetes* by Cyrus Khambata PhD and Robby Barbaro, MPH, both Type 1 Diabetics. This book is very informative for Type 1 and Type 2 Diabetics.

Day 15: **YOUR HEART TO SOUL DAILY JOURNAL**

DATE: _____

DAILY WEIGHT: _____ **A.M. GLUCOSE:** _____

TODAY'S OVERALL FEELING OF WELLNESS:

1   2   3   4   5   6   7   8   9   10

INTENTION WORD FOR THE DAY: _____

TODAY I ACCOMPLISHED:

☐ Mindful breath work

☐ Mindful meditation (Duration _____)

☐ Joy & Meaning self-care activity: _____

3 THINGS I AM GRATEFUL FOR TODAY:

1.

2.

3.

WHAT'S ON YOUR MIND?

Day 16: YOUR HEART TO SOUL DAILY JOURNAL

DATE: _____

DAILY WEIGHT:_____ A.M. GLUCOSE:_____

TODAY'S OVERALL FEELING OF WELLNESS:

1   2   3   4   5   6   7   8   9   10

INTENTION WORD FOR THE DAY:_____

TODAY I ACCOMPLISHED:

☐ Mindful breath work

☐ Mindful meditation (Duration _____)

☐ Joy & Meaning self-care activity:_____

3 THINGS I AM GRATEFUL FOR TODAY:

1.

2.

3.

WHAT'S ON YOUR MIND?

Day 17: YOUR HEART TO SOUL DAILY JOURNAL

DATE: _____

DAILY WEIGHT: _____ A.M. GLUCOSE: _____

TODAY'S OVERALL FEELING OF WELLNESS:

1   2   3   4   5   6   7   8   9   10

INTENTION WORD FOR THE DAY: _____

TODAY I ACCOMPLISHED:

☐ Mindful breath work

☐ Mindful meditation (Duration _____)

☐ Joy & Meaning self-care activity: _____

3 THINGS I AM GRATEFUL FOR TODAY:

1.

2.

3.

WHAT'S ON YOUR MIND?

Day 18: **YOUR HEART TO SOUL DAILY JOURNAL**

DATE: _____

DAILY WEIGHT: _____ **A.M. GLUCOSE:** _____

TODAY'S OVERALL FEELING OF WELLNESS:

1   2   3   4   5   6   7   8   9   10

INTENTION WORD FOR THE DAY: _____

TODAY I ACCOMPLISHED:

☐ Mindful breath work

☐ Mindful meditation (Duration _____)

☐ Joy & Meaning self-care activity: _____

3 THINGS I AM GRATEFUL FOR TODAY:

1.

2.

3.

WHAT'S ON YOUR MIND?

Day 19: YOUR HEART TO SOUL DAILY JOURNAL

DATE: _____

DAILY WEIGHT: _____   A.M. GLUCOSE: _____

TODAY'S OVERALL FEELING OF WELLNESS:

1   2   3   4   5   6   7   8   9   10

INTENTION WORD FOR THE DAY: _____

TODAY I ACCOMPLISHED:

☐ Mindful breath work

☐ Mindful meditation (Duration _____)

☐ Joy & Meaning self-care activity: _____

3 THINGS I AM GRATEFUL FOR TODAY:

1.

2.

3.

WHAT'S ON YOUR MIND?

Day 20: **YOUR HEART TO SOUL DAILY JOURNAL**

DATE: _____

DAILY WEIGHT: _____ **A.M. GLUCOSE:** _____

TODAY'S OVERALL FEELING OF WELLNESS:

1   2   3   4   5   6   7   8   9   10

INTENTION WORD FOR THE DAY: _____

TODAY I ACCOMPLISHED:

☐ Mindful breath work

☐ Mindful meditation (Duration _____)

☐ Joy & Meaning self-care activity: _____

3 THINGS I AM GRATEFUL FOR TODAY:

1.

2.

3.

WHAT'S ON YOUR MIND?

Day 21: **YOUR HEART TO SOUL DAILY JOURNAL**

DATE: _____

DAILY WEIGHT: _____   **A.M. GLUCOSE:** _____

TODAY'S OVERALL FEELING OF WELLNESS:

1   2   3   4   5   6   7   8   9   10

INTENTION WORD FOR THE DAY: _____

TODAY I ACCOMPLISHED:

☐ Mindful breath work

☐ Mindful meditation (Duration _____)

☐ Joy & Meaning self-care activity: _____

3 THINGS I AM GRATEFUL FOR TODAY:

1.

2.

3.

WHAT'S ON YOUR MIND?

Week 4:

DOES DAIRY "DO YOUR BODY GOOD"? MOO!

Dairy: Does it do your body good, as the dairy industry and marketing milk mustaches tell you? Please note: Some of the information in the next two chapters may be difficult to read. After all, we learned to love whole milk, full-fat ice cream, butter, whipped cream, sour cream and even yogurt as we grew up, thinking they were healthy. The message was milk gave us strong bones and healthy hearts. We were encouraged to eat cheese, had milk served to us at school and we picked up cheeseburgers, fries, and milkshakes for dinner.

WHAT IS SO BAD HERE, YOU MAY ASK?

Our bodies are chemistry sets, and some of the intake lab values requested in the beginning of your book were inflammatory markers. Dairy products cause disease-producing inflammation in our bodies.

Dairy and other animal products such as meat and eggs, can cause our body to go into an acidic inflammatory state. Humans normally have a balance of pH in the range of 7.35 (acidic) to 7.45 (alkaline) on a scale of 0-14. That is only a .10 differential. If our bodies are challenged by something unusual going on, they work to correct the imbalance and move back to homeostasis (our balanced state). Our bodies *want* to feel good and they have mechanisms to screen, clean, and correct things that they sense are out of their balance of homeostasis.

OUR NUTRITION IS THE BIGGEST FACTOR IN HELPING OUR BODY OPTIMIZE ITSELF.

When we eat dairy or any animal product, it can create an acidic environment. What does our body do to counteract the acidic environment? It can leach calcium from our bones to buffer the acidity. So, while we have a high amount of dairy intake in our country, we resultantly have a high rate of osteoporosis.

Milk and dairy products are a top source of saturated fat in the Standard American Diet, and have been proven to contribute to heart disease, breast and prostate cancer, Type 2 diabetes and Alzheimer's disease.

One more time with feeling! Please share this with three people you care about today: **The "Standard American Diet," which includes dairy and meat, leads to the "Standard American Diseases," which then lead to the "Standard American Medications."** Your choices of what you eat will have direct consequences affecting your health, your free time, and your wallet.

SAD SAD SAM

I am here to empower you with knowledge so that you have the ability to understand why certain foods can make you sick, so that you can change how and what you eat to improve your health. We don't have to eat the Standard American Diet. We can change our nutritional intake to healing foods like legumes, grains, vegetables and fruits to promote health and enable our immune systems to fight diseases. We can "Live our life on the Veg!"

A perfect example of a patient who turned her life around simply by turning her nutrition around was "Abbie" (not her real name). Abbie had been my patient in the hospital, having survived a heart attack. About five months after her hospitalization, Abbie saw me walking in Washington Square Park and she ran (ran!) up to me with a big smile on her face, waving her hand to me while calling out "Nurse Mary, Nurse Mary, it's me, Abbie!" I did not recognize her because she looked so much healthier than when I took care of her at the hospital. She had lost a lot of weight, which made her feel confident about herself and she had started to exercise, which made her feel stronger in her body. She said she had moved to eating vegetarian and was loving it because she felt so much better, and she was excited to be learning how to make simple yet tasty healthy meals. Her goal was to become vegan by eliminating eggs and dairy from her meals, as she had recently read information about the heart health benefits of eliminating all meats and eggs and dairy from the foods you eat. Abbie had done great work and she started by simply making small changes, one meal at a time and one walk around the block at a time.

Before these changes, Abbie had been in love with the wrong foods, which led to her heart attack.

Remember how we talked about foods we culturally learned to love, and how it was really difficult for my friend to separate himself from his mozzarella? What we have developed is a culture and habit of eating foods that were not meant for us. We have developed brain connections wired to memories of sitting at dinners for occasions, such as holidays, family BBQs, and birthday celebrations. Food has indeed become intertwined with how we relate and make associations, but not necessarily in the best interest of our health. The "family history" of BBQs, steak dinners, crab boils, and tons of butter might be causing the "family history" of heart disease. It is important to understand this concept of our family history, traditions, and culture in relation to our health and disease processes. To make the changes needed for our health, it is necessary to change our mind regarding the way we see our food. We have eaten a certain way because that is what we are used to, and what has happened over time is that we as a nation have gotten sicker and sicker.

The CDC reports that in 1960, national health expenditures on prescription drugs was 2.7 billion dollars. In 2017 it was 333.4 billion dollars. That is over 123 times an increase in 57 years!

> **Might it be a conflict of interest that the same government body oversees and regulates BOTH food and drugs?**

Might this be how "The Standard American Diet" leads to "The Standard American Diseases" which leads to "The Standard American Medications" we see advertised on TV, right after an advertisement for the type of food that *causes* the illness that this drug "helps"? Consider a commercial for pizza followed by four commercials; one for a heart disease medication, one for a "lactose intolerance" medication, a third medication to calm an upset stomach and a fourth about a cancer center. Do healthy people make any of these drug companies or the cancer center money? No, but the Standard American Diet—including meat and dairy—sure does help these industries to prosper.

> **Healthy people don't make money for these companies— sick people do. Consider who is making profits when you *first* spend the money to purchase and eat animal products and contrived food products and *then* after you acquire an illness because of eating this way.**

I remember a conversation I had with a patient who had survived a heart attack, and we were discussing how meat and dairy can contribute to cardiac disease. I left his room to attend to another patient, and a few minutes later, his call bell went off. I went back into his room to ask him what he needed. He said he couldn't eat his lunch and he pointed to his lunch tray that had just been delivered. I looked down at the tray and there it was, a hamburger and milk, served in the cardiac unit to a patient who had a heart attack. Doesn't this speak volumes about SAD SAD SAM? The patient requested to change his meals to vegan instead of the standard diet offered in the hospital, which he now knew would make him sick again.

I am pleased to share that in New York, plant-based options are now on hospital menus, and the New York City hospitals and schools observe "Meatless Monday" meal service.

Unfortunately, there is *not* a lot of information in ads about holistic disease prevention and health optimization; things like eating a green, a bean and a fruit at each meal, exercising, and what stress relief can do for your heart and greater health. That is why we are here together, now.

As I was speaking with Abbie, I reflected back to the brief conversation I had with her in the hospital, because she had been so despondent. In that conversation, I had encouraged Abbie that while she had a heart attack, she was safe, the emergent interventional procedure that had been done on her had helped her, and that she could make lifestyle changes like minimizing or removing dairy and meat from the foods she ate to protect her future health. Abbie thanked me for taking care of her and being kind to her. I walked away from our conversation at her bedside in the hospital that day feeling so honored that I was able to say something that would help Abbie to make positive health changes that would affect how she approached life anew.

We never know what single thing we might say or do may have such a great life-changing impact on someone. The good news is that like Abbie, we are capable of creating new cultures and traditions from making healthier food choices. You can do it, too!

- -

"KNOWING IS NOT ENOUGH, WE MUST APPLY.
WILLING IS NOT ENOUGH, WE MUST DO."
—**BRUCE LEE,** martial artist, actor, philosopher

- -

NOW, LET'S GET TO THE BOTTOM OF THE GLASS OF MILK

Why else is dairy scary and what else is going on ethically and morally with the sourcing of animal products that brings them onto our plates and into our glass?

Reflection Questions: Why don't we give newborn infants cow's milk, and instead give them only breast milk or formula? Why are people taking medications for "lactose intolerance?"

Lactose intolerance is the inability of the body to break down the sugar in dairy products called lactose. Milk from any species is only meant for the newborn offspring of that species, to feed them high nutrition so they can grow and provide natural immunity to protect them from illness. All of these animals, including humans, are naturally weaned by their mothers. The mother's milk is necessary for the species infant's initial growth and immunity, but is not required after weaning. *Adults of any species are not supposed to drink milk because nature only meant for it to be a starter food!* The ability of the body to process lactose is lost after weaning time for this reason!

"YOU CAN'T EXPECT TO FEEL LIKE A MILLION BUCKS IF YOU EAT DAIRY; WHAT YOU CAN EXPECT IS DIGESTIVE PROBLEMS."

—ANGIE SADEGHI, MD, board certified gastroenterologist,

Author, *The Trifecta of Health*

Not everyone may exhibit lactose intolerance, or they may not connect that their symptoms such as gas, bloating, abdominal cramps or diarrhea are a result of lactose intolerance; but everyone is susceptible to diseases such as heart disease and cancer, caused by eating and drinking dairy products. We are "lactose intolerant" because we are supposed to be. Lactose intolerance is nature's way of saying "This is not meant for you!"

Reflection Questions: Does it make sense to take a medication for "lactose intolerance" when by nature, we are not meant to eat or drink dairy or its "products," especially from another species? How might someone be "playing themselves" by taking a pill every time they have dairy or else they feel ill? How are they setting themselves up for heart disease, diabetes, cancer, and other illnesses? It is no coincidence that heart disease, diabetes, and cancer are in the top ten causes for mortality in the United States.

We don't give a human infant the milk from another species such as a cow because it contains hormones and growth factors such as IGF-1. Cow's milk is chemically designed with hormones by nature for the purpose of nurturing and rapidly growing a bovine: a baby cow, *not* a human infant. Cows make milk as a natural byproduct of giving birth; it is their lactation, their "breast milk," from *their* udder for *their* newborn, not for a human. Cow's milk has been known to make human babies sick because they are unable to process it in their system. In an article written for The Natural Child Project, Linda Folden, D.C. (Doctor of Chiropractic) illuminates "The Dangers of Cow's Milk." "Cow's milk is a foreign substance that has pervaded every corner of our diets—starting with artificial infant feeds, but finding its way into mother's breastmilk through the food she eats as well. As it turns out, health problems such as childhood diabetes, obesity, bowel disease, osteoporosis, heart disease, cataracts, colic, ear infections, hyperactivity and cancer, on the rise in both children and adults, can be strongly linked to infant feeding choices."

From what you have learned so far about dairy, what do you think of these ingredients I found on an infant formula label:

- Nonfat milk (cow's milk)
- Vegetable oil (oil as the second ingredient with more oils to follow)
- Lactose (cow's milk)
- Whey protein (cow's milk)
- Galactooligosaccharides (sugar)
- Polydextrose (a synthetic lab-made glucose polymer)
- Mortierella alpina oil
- Crypthecodinium cohnii oil

This list goes on and includes some vitamins. What do you think about this list? Would you want to have this as your sole source of nutrition the first months of your life? Might we possibly have babies labeled as suffering from "colic" when they may be suffering from the ingredients of their formula?

"YOU SHOULDN'T BE DRINKING COW'S MILK FOR THE SAME REASON THAT IF YOU NEED A BLOOD TRANSFUSION, I WOULDN'T GIVE YOU COW'S BLOOD. IT'S NOT MEANT FOR A HUMAN."

—DR. MILTON MILLS, Associate Director of Preventive Medicine for the Physicians Committee for Responsible Medicine (PCRM)

Dr. T. Colin Campbell, an American biochemist who specializes in the effect of nutrition on long-term health and Professor Emeritus of Nutritional Biochemistry at Cornell University, reports from his research that there is a link between the protein called casein in dairy to breast and prostate cancers. Dr. Campbell researched and wrote about this link extensively in his book *The China Study*. Now, take casein, a carcinogen, and combine it with IGF-1 growth factor, a protein produced by the liver which could make cancer grow more rapidly. This makes dairy a dangerous toxic food! Casein, and its chemical derivative caseinate are hidden in a lot of food products. Cheese (which contains casein) has been proven to be addictive because our bodies convert casein to casomorphin, an addicting compound in the same chemical family as morphine and opium. It stimulates our pleasure centers in our brain. Is this possibly why casein and its derivatives are added into food products by food scientists—to get us to buy more and eat more?

"CASEIN IS THE MOST RELEVANT CHEMICAL CARCINOGEN EVER IDENTIFIED."

—DR. T. COLIN CAMPBELL, Professor Emeritus of Nutritional Biochemistry at Cornell University.

Cheese is concentrated fat: that's why it tastes good to us. Think of taking many pounds of milk and its fat content and condensing it down to that package of butter or cheese that you see in the supermarket. What happens to our arteries when we eat foods containing fat? Where does that fat go? It goes into our artery walls and our cells. Recall "Fat" the bouncer who was at the cell "club," causing an increase in diabetes.

As you are now aware, dairy is toxic to our bodies. We can find the calcium we need in foods like fruits and vegetables. The Physicians Committee for Responsible Medicine is demanding that the newly released USDA 2020-2025 Dietary Guidelines be retracted and reworked to delete dairy promotion, avoid equating "protein" with meat, and increase emphasis on plant-based foods.

> **The takeaway here is this: We don't need dairy to get the calcium we need.**

Let's pull back the curtain to see what is going on behind the scenes in the dairy industry, morally and ethically, so we can be informed in what we chose to be on our plate and in our cells. What was the sourcing of your dairy products? How did humans get another species' lactation (milk) in our grocery stores and onto our tables at home and in our schools? Again, some of this material may be difficult to read. However, the information presented here is for you to be able to make new choices as a result of your knowledge.

On a dairy farm, the female cows are impregnated artificially by humans physically depositing sperm into them that was taken from a male cow, a bull. After giving birth, the babies are immediately taken from their mothers. It is believed that the mother is in a state of grieving and trauma, as is the baby cow. On large dairy farms, not long after birth, each baby girl cow is placed in an individual pen and bottle-fed formula. Remember, the money making business here is milk, and the mother's milk is going into milk machines and to your table, not to the baby cow. If these babies will not drink, they are force-fed the formula with a tube down their throat. Truck drivers drive down rows of animals and plop a large container of formula with a nipple on it onto the fence that pens in the baby. They feed off that bottle. They are not socialized with their mother or in groups on these large dairy farms; they are individually penned and live in little igloo-like structures for shelter. On some small farms, if they are allowed to socialize, the babies' noses are pierced with a spiked ring so if they do try to take milk from the mother's udder, the spikes will cause pain and she will move away. The milk is for the machines and the dairy industry, not for the mother and her baby. A mother cow is impregnated again, her baby taken again and possibly for another time or two, so long as her body can produce. Imagine if you went through pregnancy, delivered your baby, got to see it, then had it taken away, repeatedly, pregnancy after pregnancy, and you were hooked up to machines many times a day. These cows must be in a perpetual state of grief.

A baby boy calf is of no use to the dairy industry and most of them will be killed and sold as veal.

The grieving and traumatized new mother is placed on milking machines that take her milk, sometimes even before she gives birth, while she is still pregnant and starting to develop milk. Some farmers give these cows hormones that make the size of their udder painfully large to produce even more milk for more profit. These cows get infections, and are placed on antibiotics, which are passed on to you in their flesh and milk. The pus from the infection goes in the milk, which is one reason why it is cooked (pasteurized) prior to packaging. This cycle of impregnation and taking the baby so she can be a milk-producing machine happens repeatedly for a female dairy cow, until her body is spent, in about 4-5 cycles or 6 years, when she would normally live upwards of 20 years in nature. When she can no longer produce milk sufficiently, her worn out body is made into ground meat. When I see a dairy farm now, I think of it as a place of immense sadness, grief, and torture.

These cows may develop sores and tumors in and on their bodies. Is anyone doing surgery on animals to remove abscesses and tumors from any animal before its flesh is ground up to become your hamburger, wings, or steak on your plate? No—it is all going into the mix. Hundreds of disease-ridden cows may comprise your single hamburger patty. Cows live in their excrement, and this is why we have meat supplies and farmland nearby infected with their E. coli fecal bacteria.

How does this dead flesh translate into helping your cells and body thrive? It doesn't. It puts you at risk for food borne diseases, heart disease, diabetes, and obesity. This is not food, it is dead flesh and serves as a stamp on our passport to the "Cardiac Bermuda Triangle."

These farm animals are raised in barns with minimal land, and fed cheap GMO corn and soy. Remember what the animal eats is in its flesh and you are resultantly ingesting it. GMOs are Genetically Modified Organisms, meaning that through science, the natural product was altered, perhaps to be able to grow and thrive in an herbicide, so when the plants are sprayed with this toxin, they can still grow in it. By nature, cows largely feed on grass. Herbicide and pesticide-drenched genetically modified soy and corn (not their natural food) crops for animals take up land space that could be used for our own human crops. The topsoil is polluted with pesticides. The area is polluted with excrement, and the runoff from the pesticides and feces kills fish and wildlife in our rivers and streams, and ultimately goes into the ocean, killing more fish. The Earth's atmosphere is damaged by the methane gas these animals pass as flatulence, which has contributed to global warming more than any other industry.

Consider that culturally in the Western world, we do not eat cats and dogs, but they are eaten in other countries and used as a commodity just as we have commodified animals such as cows, pigs, sheep, chickens, turkeys, and goats. We would be outraged if we saw a dog or cat on a grill in a backyard. Yet we do this with these other animals that have feelings and bonds with their families and friends. How is this kind of factory farming negatively impacting our health, these animals, our environment, our crops, and the sustainability of the Earth? What are the politics behind what we eat?

ZOONOTIC DISEASES

At the time of this writing, in the fall of 2020, we are combating the pandemic of the COVID-19 virus. Consider the cause and origination of the following diseases, which have directly made humans sick. These disease origins were zoonotic, meaning that they were transferred from animal to human. These human diseases ALL originated from eating, or contact with, diseased animals.

Zoonotic diseases include the following:

- SARS virus from bats to civet cats

- MERS virus from camel meat

- CARDIAC DISEASE animal meat and dairy products

- CANCER animal meat and dairy products

- NIPAH virus from pig meat

- HIV virus from chimpanzee meat

- AVIAN FLU virus from bird meat

- H1N1 Swine flu virus from pig meat

- E. COLI from cow meat and excrement

- MAD COW DISEASE from cow meat

- SALMONELLA from chicken and reptile meat

- TRICHINOSIS from pig meat

- PARASITES AND WORMS from animal flesh

- FOOD POISONING from animal flesh

"MAJOR COMORBIDITY CONDITIONS FOR COVID-19 SEVERITY AND DEATH ARE OBESITY, HEART DISEASE, HYPERTENSION AND TYPE 2 DIABETES—ALL OF WHICH MAY ALL BE CONTROLLED OR EVEN REVERSED WITH A HEALTHY PLANT-BASED DIET."

—DR. MICHAEL GREGER, plant-based nutrition expert, author

The risk for diseases, like heart disease, or a pandemic illness far outweighs the reward of a passing sensation on your taste buds. Is that piece of steak or bacon worth increasing your health risk? Is it kind to the animal? What is the risk versus the reward of eating it?

> **Dairy does not seem to do a body good, does it?**
> **(Cows that were polled with this question answered "Moo!")**

Remember that like Abbie did, taking small steps toward better health is all it takes to start on a path that will lead to better health. After all, many of us were raised on butter, cheese, meat, and milk. Change will take conscious thoughtfulness, time, and will be incremental. It doesn't have to be overnight. What matters is that you're making strides toward better health now.

"DON'T BE SO HARD ON YOURSELF! AS PERFECT AS WE LIKE TO THINK WE ARE, YOU WILL MESS UP. THE KEY IS NOT TO BEAT YOURSELF UP ABOUT IT. IF YOU SLIP UP AND EAT CHEESE AT 11:59 MAKE SURE YOU ARE RIGHT BACK ON THE PATH AT 12:00. DON'T WASTE TIME BEATING YOURSELF UP BECAUSE OF THAT MISTAKE. GET RIGHT BACK ON THE PATH TO A HEALTHIER LIFESTYLE!"

—JOHN LEWIS, aka the "Badass Vegan," and

Filmmaker, *They're Trying to Kill Us*

PRO TIP: There are plant-based yogurts, cheeses, and other alternatives to explore. Your neighborhood supermarket may not have them and you may need to look for a health food store, but the good news is there are more and more mainstream non-dairy options coming to the marketplace. Check out the organic aisle in your supermarket. Once you find substitutes you enjoy, you will be able to "wean" off of dairy. Your arteries will be cheering you on! Your taste buds will jump for joy, too, once they "see" how great these foods are!

PRO TIP: If you are going to a restaurant, let's say for pizza, you can pick the cheese off, or better yet, order your pizza with red sauce and vegetables. Spice it up with oregano and red pepper flakes. Maybe you could even kick up the healthiness a bit further and try a gluten-free crust!

PRO TIP: Oat milk is a better alternative than almond milk because of the large amounts of water required to grow almonds. There are some consciously aware coffee shops that charge for almond milk, and offer oat milk or soy milk free as encouragement for environmental protection and awareness.

> **PRO TIP**: As much as possible, select USDA ORGANIC and NON-GMO (Genetically Modified Organisms) for your food choices.

Let's start setting goals today to change our cultural behaviors and rituals to new, healthy ones. If you want to get to better health, it is necessary to change what you are doing here and now.

GOAL:

I will thoughtfully begin to eliminate dairy from the foods I eat. My ultimate goal is that by the end of the 66th day in my accountability agreement, I will not eat dairy because I now know how bad dairy is for me, that it is not meant for me, and that I will be saving animals' lives, while helping the planet.

WEEKLY HOMEWORK
(CHECK OFF WHEN COMPLETED)

☐ Locate, try out, and share with others new non-dairy options in place of dairy.

☐ Experiment with different non-dairy plant based milk alternatives. There are so many options to replace dairy milk: rice milk, cashew milk, oat milk, flax milk, hemp milk, almond milk, soy milk, and even banana milk! Over time, your tastes will change and you will be supported in the knowledge that you are making adjustments that will positively impact your health. The shift is from an "I can't have this" mindset to an "I could have this, but I am choosing not to, because it is not good for me. I want to add years to my life, and life in those years" mindset.

☐ Read "The Dangers of Cow's Milk." By Linda Folden, D.C. online

☐ Watch the movie *Earthlings* (2005). It can be found online.

☐ Watch the movie *Cowspiracy* (2014) online.

Day 22: **YOUR HEART TO SOUL DAILY JOURNAL**

DATE: _____

DAILY WEIGHT: _____ **A.M. GLUCOSE:** _____

TODAY'S OVERALL FEELING OF WELLNESS:

1   2   3   4   5   6   7   8   9   10

INTENTION WORD FOR THE DAY: _____

TODAY I ACCOMPLISHED:

☐ Mindful breath work

☐ Mindful meditation (Duration _____)

☐ Joy & Meaning self-care activity: _____

3 THINGS I AM GRATEFUL FOR TODAY:

1.

2.

3.

WHAT'S ON YOUR MIND?

Day 23: **YOUR HEART TO SOUL DAILY JOURNAL**

DATE: _____

DAILY WEIGHT: _____ **A.M. GLUCOSE:** _____

TODAY'S OVERALL FEELING OF WELLNESS:

1   2   3   4   5   6   7   8   9   10

INTENTION WORD FOR THE DAY: _____

TODAY I ACCOMPLISHED:

☐ Mindful breath work

☐ Mindful meditation (Duration _____)

☐ Joy & Meaning self-care activity: _____

3 THINGS I AM GRATEFUL FOR TODAY:

1.

2.

3.

WHAT'S ON YOUR MIND?

Day 24: YOUR HEART TO SOUL DAILY JOURNAL

DATE: _____

DAILY WEIGHT: _____   **A.M. GLUCOSE:** _____

TODAY'S OVERALL FEELING OF WELLNESS:

1   2   3   4   5   6   7   8   9   10

INTENTION WORD FOR THE DAY: _____

TODAY I ACCOMPLISHED:

☐ Mindful breath work

☐ Mindful meditation (Duration _____)

☐ Joy & Meaning self-care activity: _____

3 THINGS I AM GRATEFUL FOR TODAY:

1.

2.

3.

WHAT'S ON YOUR MIND?

Day 25: **YOUR HEART TO SOUL DAILY JOURNAL**

DATE: _____

DAILY WEIGHT: _____ **A.M. GLUCOSE:** _____

TODAY'S OVERALL FEELING OF WELLNESS:

1   2   3   4   5   6   7   8   9   10

INTENTION WORD FOR THE DAY: _____

TODAY I ACCOMPLISHED:

☐ Mindful breath work

☐ Mindful meditation (Duration _____)

☐ Joy & Meaning self-care activity: _____

3 THINGS I AM GRATEFUL FOR TODAY:

1.

2.

3.

WHAT'S ON YOUR MIND?

Day 26: **YOUR HEART TO SOUL DAILY JOURNAL**

DATE: _____

DAILY WEIGHT: _____ **A.M. GLUCOSE:** _____

TODAY'S OVERALL FEELING OF WELLNESS:

1   2   3   4   5   6   7   8   9   10

INTENTION WORD FOR THE DAY: _____

TODAY I ACCOMPLISHED:

☐ Mindful breath work

☐ Mindful meditation (Duration _____)

☐ Joy & Meaning self-care activity: _____

3 THINGS I AM GRATEFUL FOR TODAY:

1.

2.

3.

WHAT'S ON YOUR MIND?

Day 27: YOUR HEART TO SOUL DAILY JOURNAL

DATE: _____

DAILY WEIGHT:_____ A.M. GLUCOSE:_____

TODAY'S OVERALL FEELING OF WELLNESS:

1   2   3   4   5   6   7   8   9   10

INTENTION WORD FOR THE DAY:_____

TODAY I ACCOMPLISHED:

☐ Mindful breath work

☐ Mindful meditation (Duration _____)

☐ Joy & Meaning self-care activity:_____

3 THINGS I AM GRATEFUL FOR TODAY:

1.

2.

3.

WHAT'S ON YOUR MIND?

Day 28: YOUR HEART TO SOUL DAILY JOURNAL

DATE: _____

DAILY WEIGHT: _____   A.M. GLUCOSE: _____

TODAY'S OVERALL FEELING OF WELLNESS:

1   2   3   4   5   6   7   8   9   10

INTENTION WORD FOR THE DAY: _____

TODAY I ACCOMPLISHED:

☐ Mindful breath work

☐ Mindful meditation (Duration _____)

☐ Joy & Meaning self-care activity: _____

3 THINGS I AM GRATEFUL FOR TODAY:

1.

2.

3.

WHAT'S ON YOUR MIND?

Week 5:
CHEWING THE FAT ABOUT MEAT

How are we doing so far? This has been a lot of information to process. How are you feeling after minimizing or not eating dairy for a week? Does your mind feel clearer? Have you brought anyone along with you on your journey? Take a moment to reflect on your accountability agreement. How does your accountability partner in the bathroom mirror look and feel today?

I want to tell you that you are doing a great job at putting in the effort here. I realize that much of this is new. Take it easy, one bite at a time.

Let's chew the fat about meat and talk about protein. Where do we get our protein if we do not eat meat? Does a rhino eat steaks and burgers? Does a gorilla? Does a rhino use a blender and supplement his smoothie with protein powder? Do cows eat other animals? If the answer to all of these questions is "No," then how the heck do cows and rhinos get their protein? They get their protein from plants!

A rhino is an herbivore—nature's vegan. A vegan is a person who eats plants. Vegans do not eat any animal products or byproducts, including eggs and butter or products containing them such as baked goods or candy. Some vegans have even incorporated veganism into their lifestyle, removing leather items from their wardrobe and home. These are options to consider, but by no means am I suggesting that you throw out your favorite shoes and purses because they are leather. When you are ready to purchase new things, there are some fun, hip, on-trend companies offering products that are eco-friendly, sustainable, harmless to animals, and less expensive, too! If you do choose to move into a plant based (and planet-based) vegan lifestyle, you will find there is a whole new world of resources, support and a really genuine and passionate community of people ready to help you, and to cheer you on!

Back to this week's topic. So… let's think about this: Does a rhino look frail or malnourished? Have you ever heard of a vegan unit in a hospital for sick, protein deficient vegans? Have you heard of a cardiac intensive care unit in a hospital? Of course. The cardiac units are some of the busiest units in hospitals. That's because cardiac disease is the number one cause of death in the U.S, and it has been for over eighty years. Have you ever heard of a protein deficiency unit in the hospital because people aren't eating enough protein? No, but there are dialysis units and dialysis centers to care for kidney patients. One of the contributors to kidney disease can be intake of excess protein. For example, if someone eats a bacon egg and cheese sandwich for breakfast with a glass of milk, a burger at lunch with a shake and chicken wings and steak for dinner, we are already talking about a lot of protein on the plate before we have even considered the protein in any vegetables, beans or other foods they may have consumed that day. Eating many foods high in proteins like animal products, protein bars, protein shakes, and protein powder assaults the kidneys with a burden they cannot process. This problem is made worse for the kidneys if the person has hypertension and/or is diabetic. Consider the source of a protein: a dead animal or a plant, like beans. Which choice if put on the end of your fork, is going to be healthier for your body?

"LET'S TAKE A WALK IN THE COUNTRY!"

Let's compare our refrigerated meat counter in the supermarket with a walk in the country. Let's say you are walking down a country road on a winter day. It is 38 degrees Fahrenheit out. Unfortunately, a wild turkey runs in front of a car that is passing by, and the turkey is killed, and flung into the grass at the side of the road. Each day you walk by the turkey. After three days, you see the turkey still lying there. The temperature did not ever get above 38 degrees, and there were no bugs or rodents that touched this turkey. Would you take it home to eat it? Of course not.

When we go to the grocery store, we see meat on the shelves that came from animals who were killed days before. We are looking at a dead piece of flesh that has been sitting in the refrigerator to temporarily safeguard its ultimate demise. How can eating dead flesh be healthy? What happens to this decaying flesh once it is in the heat of your 98.6 degree intestines? Meats contain cholesterol, fat and diseases like Salmonella and E. coli. How can eating something dead and possibly diseased promote your vitality?

Most of the animals raised to be exploited and killed for food are genetically modified to grow faster and bigger for quicker and higher profits. These animals are fed pesticide and herbicide-drenched and genetically modified feed crops. Each animal is pumped with drugs and supplements to boost growth in weight abnormally quickly, and to prevent infection. If we eat that animal flesh, we are indirectly taking in these toxins. Animal products labeled "organic," "pasture raised" and "grass-fed" should be avoided also, because they are still sources of cholesterol, animal hormones, protein and unhealthy fats, which have negative impacts on cardiovascular and overall health, clogging our arteries and adding to fat in the cells, creating insulin resistance.

Products from sea creatures, such as fish and fish oils, are just like the animal products from exploited land animals. Because of the way some fishing is done, by dragging nets on the sea bottom, many other sea animals such as dolphins are caught and killed, not just the type of fish being fished. Farm-raised fish are fed GMO "food pellets," and confined in antibiotic filled tanks and sometimes even have colorings added to their food to make their flesh red or pink. I encourage you to do your own research about how fish, chickens, pigs, beef, and dairy animals are raised and treated, so you know where your food was sourced and how it came to be in the supermarket.

LET'S TALK ABOUT CHOLESTEROL

Howard Lyman was a guest on Oprah Winfrey's talk show, *Dangerous Food*, which was broadcast on April 16, 1996, and featured a discussion about how cows are handled and the propensity for Mad

Cow Disease. Alarmed, Oprah asked her audience, "Now, doesn't that concern you all a little bit right there, hearing that? It has just stopped me cold from eating another burger. I'm stopped."

"JUST AS SOME PEOPLE BELIEVE THAT THEY ARE CONDEMNED TO HEART DISEASE BY BAD GENES, OTHERS ARE SO CERTAIN THAT THEIR HEALTH IS PROTECTED BY GOOD GENES THAT THEY DON'T WORRY ABOUT THE ILL EFFECTS OF EATING HIGH-CHOLESTEROL FOODS."

—HOWARD F. LYMAN, former cattle rancher,

animal rights activist, environmentalist, author

Lyman and Winfrey were both sued by a group of Texas Cattlemen. Isn't there something wrong here if you learn facts about a "food," causing you to make a statement that concerns saving your own life and then you are sued? This shows the power of these industries, and they exist because we are supporting them by buying meat. Lyman and Winfrey spent six years in court defending the truth and were vindicated. It is vital that in addition to the sourcing, you understand the politics behind your food.

Our cell membranes require cholesterol for its protective properties. Cholesterol is found in all animal products, but we do not need to add any external cholesterol into our bodies. We don't *need* meat. Our brains and bodies need cholesterol to function optimally, so the brain and liver make their own cholesterol to support our body. How cool is that?

Cholesterol is one of the reasons we get heart disease. There are two types of cholesterol: Low Density Lipoprotein (LDL), the "bad" cholesterol that sticks to our artery walls, the smaller particles being like hard little rocks, and the High-Density Lipoprotein (HDL) cholesterol, the "good" cholesterol our cells and brains need.

We recorded our beginning cholesterol labs at the start of our journey. When you first started this book, you might have been eating meat, cheese, and other foods that caused a line with "Fat," the bouncer at the entrance of the cell club. By eliminating these foods—even slowly—you're opening yourself up to improved health and clearing the way for feeling much better, because you have eliminated the line at the club, "Fat" the bouncer is gone and your cells can get their glucose and nutrient fuel. (Update: "Fat" got a new job making smoothies at a Natural Food Store in NYC! He loves it! He became vegan and lost a lot of weight, has a new girlfriend, and he feels fantastic.)

LET'S TALK ABOUT TMAO

TMAO: I wish this mnemonic stood for "Thanks, Mom, All OK!" TMAO (Trimethylamine-N-Oxide) is not something you hear about on the news, or in casual discussion anywhere, (unless you are a gastroenterologist or a cardiologist!), and I feel it is important for you to know about it and how it can affect your cholesterol levels.

TMAO is produced by our gut bacteria when we eat egg yolks and red meat. TMAO assists the development of plaque on blood vessel walls, creating greater compounded risk for heart disease. Heart disease is caused not only from what we are eating, but also in how our body processes it, in this case with egg yolks and red meat. People who have higher levels of TMAO have a higher risk of heart disease, heart attack, or stroke. People who have adopted more of a plant based heart-healthy nutrition lifestyle reduce TMAO levels.

We can see here how heart disease, diabetes, and obesity link up to form a "Bermuda Triangle of Illness." We now know that by eliminating fats, meats, dairy, fatty food products, and processed sugar, we can improve a Type 2 diabetic condition and possibly reverse it, as Eric Adams (current Brooklyn, New York, Borough President) inspiringly shares his own story in his book: *Healthy at Last*. Remember that fats block off the ability of insulin to work to let glucose in the cells. If we layer on another level of sugar to the problem, such as sugary sodas and cookies and candies, we have created thick sludgy blood, and what are we setting ourselves up for? A heart attack and diabetes. It is called "junk food" for good reason!

Think about the guy who continues to eat his breakfast of bacon, egg, and cheese sandwiches, has a burger, fries, and soda for lunch, and then a steak dinner and thinks he is "good" because he is taking cardiac medications, a statin for his elevated cholesterol, and an aspirin every day. How might he be "playing himself?"

This brings to mind "Mr. Ain't Happening." Mr. Ain't Happening refuses to give up dairy and meats, ("It ain't happening!") and clutches his pint of ice cream every night as he sits in his recliner flipping through TV channels on his remote. He continues to eat these products despite chronic arthritic knee and joint pain, inflammation, stomach problems from "lactose intolerance" and heart disease from blocked arteries, with a borderline kidney problem. He takes heart medications for cholesterol and blood pressure, medications for his kidneys, medication for arthritis and "lactose intolerance," yet he still continues to have aches and pains. On top of all this, he has erectile dysfunction. Is it any wonder that Mr. Ain't Happening is grumpy all the time? He never feels healthy because he hasn't stopped eating the foods that are making him sick, and the pills aren't helping him get better either; they are maintaining the "status quo." He cannot enjoy ice skating anymore because his knees hurt from inflammation and arthritis and he cannot play with his grandkids like he wants to. Are those food products worth that loss of vitality in his life?

A pill will not address all other factors contributing to a body-wide disease process. Our lifestyle and how we manage it, from nutrition, sleep, exercise, stress management, and social relationships, all determine the state of our health. As I heard Preventive Cardiologist Dr. Joel Kahn say in a lecture at a plant-based conference in New York City: "Prevent, don't stent!" Your disease process(es) may be reversed, even cured, but it is up to you and your actions to make that happen. Your body wants to be in its optimal natural healthy state of homeostasis, but it needs your help.

"NOT EVERYTHING THAT IS FACED CAN BE CHANGED;
BUT NOTHING CAN BE CHANGED UNTIL IT IS FACED."
—JAMES BALDWIN, novelist, playwright, activist

Stop and consider: What you resist will persist until you reconcile it. Resisting or avoiding something can turn into stress, which manifests in your body into somatic things like muscle stiffness, headaches, and pain. Over time, if this discordant feeling is not reconciled, the issues become locked into the tissues. An example of this bodily reflection of a mental conflict could be that your shoulders are always stiff, sore, and elevated to just below your earlobes. Your emotions are energy in motion, (e-motion) and if they are forced down and avoided, they can manifest also in unhealthy emotional reactions when you are triggered. The physical symptoms will not go away if the energetic and emotional issues are not addressed. This energy flow affects every facet of your life. Think about when you encounter someone in a bad mood or you see people arguing. How does that energy "feel"? You may never have paused to consider or have been aware of the energy surrounding you. Take the rest of today to begin your mindfulness journey on tapping into what your body is feeling with your own energy, and observing the energy surrounding you. Begin to fill your life with those things and people that bring you positivity, and release things that are not uplifting you.

Notice if you are having an aversion about something, which is the beginning of resisting. Consider why you are resisting. Is this something that is negative for you, or necessary and you are avoiding it? How can you come to confront it peacefully and reconcile it for yourself?

For example, you may be resisting making life changes, and want to be a "Ms. Ain't Happening," even though you are aware of information that tells you other healthier opportunities to engage in are available for you. Take this information and thread it through other areas of your life. What are you resisting? Is it causing you an internal mental conflict? Do you feel the conflict manifesting in your body? Remember your body is your friend and to get back to homeostasis, it needs you to be healthy in your emotional state, your beliefs, your relationships, your choices, self-enhancement, and self-care.

Take a few minutes, go to the website www.meat.org and watch the brief video on the homepage narrated by the famous Beatle, Paul McCartney. Please note: This video is very graphic, and shows what happens to animals to get to our plate on our table. Understanding this process is a step toward reinforcing how we can be catalyzed to make change. You cannot un-ring a bell, and you cannot un-see and be un-aware of this reality for animals once you have watched it.

> Any progress is some progress that counts as movement forward for your health, ethically for animals, and for the health of our planet. I want to encourage your "compassionate compliance" not only for yourself, but for other beings too.

PRO TIP: Some vegan dairy (and meat) alternative products like vegan meat patties may have almost or as much fat as dairy and meat products because they are made with oils. While they are better to eat than meat, it is best to enjoy these in moderation, and select (or create) vegetable options such as a bean or quinoa burger when possible. Check the ingredient and nutrition labels on these foods for fat content.

Chapter Goal: As much as possible, I will eliminate animal products from the foods I eat. I know that eating animals can make me sick, and put me at risk for diabetes, heart disease, cancer, food contamination, and other diseases. I will be helping the planet heal and save animals' lives by not eating any animal products.

WEEKLY HOMEWORK
(CHECK OFF WHEN COMPLETED)

☐ Watch the Meat.org trailer on www.meat.org

☐ Watch the movie *Fat, Sick, and Nearly Dead* (2010). It can be found online.

☐ **Read Part Three of this book:** Read the *Pre-Op: Preparing For Your Heart Surgery* chapter of this book for great takeaways if you, or someone you know needs to prepare for *any* surgery. Then, read the chapter *Post-Op: Recovering From Your Heart Surgery*, especially noting the information about depression, and about positive affirmations. Read the *What To Expect If You Are A Partner/Spouse/Caregiver* chapter for takeaways for support in the event you need assume a caregiver role. There are tips in this chapter you can use anytime for anyone, and I want you to know this support is available for you to call upon. **Next, read the chapter about CPR.**

☐ Close your eyes for a moment and send all cardiac surgery patients everywhere some positive energy.

Day 29: **YOUR HEART TO SOUL DAILY JOURNAL**

DATE: _____

DAILY WEIGHT: _____   **A.M. GLUCOSE:** _____

TODAY'S OVERALL FEELING OF WELLNESS:

1   2   3   4   5   6   7   8   9   10

INTENTION WORD FOR THE DAY: _____

TODAY I ACCOMPLISHED:

☐ Mindful breath work

☐ Mindful meditation (Duration _____)

☐ Joy & Meaning self-care activity: _____

3 THINGS I AM GRATEFUL FOR TODAY:

1.

2.

3.

WHAT'S ON YOUR MIND?

Day 30: YOUR HEART TO SOUL DAILY JOURNAL

DATE: _____

DAILY WEIGHT: _____ **A.M. GLUCOSE:** _____

TODAY'S OVERALL FEELING OF WELLNESS:

1   2   3   4   5   6   7   8   9   10

INTENTION WORD FOR THE DAY: _____

TODAY I ACCOMPLISHED:

☐ Mindful breath work

☐ Mindful meditation (Duration _____)

☐ Joy & Meaning self-care activity: _____

3 THINGS I AM GRATEFUL FOR TODAY:

1.

2.

3.

WHAT'S ON YOUR MIND?

Day 31: YOUR HEART TO SOUL DAILY JOURNAL

DATE: _____

DAILY WEIGHT: _____   A.M. GLUCOSE: _____

TODAY'S OVERALL FEELING OF WELLNESS:

1   2   3   4   5   6   7   8   9   10

INTENTION WORD FOR THE DAY: _____

TODAY I ACCOMPLISHED:

☐ Mindful breath work

☐ Mindful meditation (Duration _____)

☐ Joy & Meaning self-care activity: _____

3 THINGS I AM GRATEFUL FOR TODAY:

1.

2.

3.

WHAT'S ON YOUR MIND?

Day 32: YOUR HEART TO SOUL DAILY JOURNAL

DATE: _____

DAILY WEIGHT: _____   A.M. GLUCOSE: _____

TODAY'S OVERALL FEELING OF WELLNESS:

1   2   3   4   5   6   7   8   9   10

INTENTION WORD FOR THE DAY: _____

TODAY I ACCOMPLISHED:

☐ Mindful breath work

☐ Mindful meditation (Duration _____)

☐ Joy & Meaning self-care activity: _____

3 THINGS I AM GRATEFUL FOR TODAY:

1.

2.

3.

WHAT'S ON YOUR MIND?

Day 33: **YOUR HEART TO SOUL DAILY JOURNAL**

DATE: _____

DAILY WEIGHT:_____   A.M. GLUCOSE:_____

TODAY'S OVERALL FEELING OF WELLNESS:

1   2   3   4   5   6   7   8   9   10

INTENTION WORD FOR THE DAY:_____

TODAY I ACCOMPLISHED:

☐ Mindful breath work

☐ Mindful meditation (Duration _____)

☐ Joy & Meaning self-care activity:_____

3 THINGS I AM GRATEFUL FOR TODAY:

1.

2.

3.

WHAT'S ON YOUR MIND?

Day 34: **YOUR HEART TO SOUL DAILY JOURNAL**

DATE: _____

DAILY WEIGHT: _____   A.M. GLUCOSE: _____

TODAY'S OVERALL FEELING OF WELLNESS:

1   2   3   4   5   6   7   8   9   10

INTENTION WORD FOR THE DAY: _____

TODAY I ACCOMPLISHED:

☐ Mindful breath work

☐ Mindful meditation (Duration _____)

☐ Joy & Meaning self-care activity: _____

3 THINGS I AM GRATEFUL FOR TODAY:

1.

2.

3.

WHAT'S ON YOUR MIND?

Day 35: YOUR HEART TO SOUL DAILY JOURNAL

DATE: _____

DAILY WEIGHT: _____   A.M. GLUCOSE: _____

TODAY'S OVERALL FEELING OF WELLNESS:

1   2   3   4   5   6   7   8   9   10

INTENTION WORD FOR THE DAY: _____

TODAY I ACCOMPLISHED:

☐ Mindful breath work

☐ Mindful meditation (Duration _____)

☐ Joy & Meaning self-care activity: _____

3 THINGS I AM GRATEFUL FOR TODAY:

1.

2.

3.

WHAT'S ON YOUR MIND?

Week 6:
LIVE YOUR LIFE ON THE VEG!

want you to know that I am the first enrollee in this *Heart to Soul Cardiac Wellness* mini boot camp! I sat in your seat, and have gathered knowledge until I had my own moment of realization. I used to think I was doing all of the right things for my body; having yogurt every day, drinking milk, eating cheese, and eating the "less fatty" meats like turkey and chicken. I did not even realize that I had a brain fog and mental slowness from dairy until I gave it up. I felt so much better without the inflammation, hormones, casein, and unnecessary additional protein and fat. I decreased my cancer risk when I gave up dairy. I understand this path you are on here and I know it can be hard to give up some foods you love, but you know what? The tradeoff in the vitality you feel and the health you obtain is worth it! I know firsthand that it is not easy to make these changes, especially when we have always thought that these foods were good for us.

Moments of friction in our lives are catalysts for change. When we get out of our comfort zone to change, we experience new things. I have found so many fantastic new brands, recipes and foods by making this shift, and I personally feel so much better. Saying "Yes" to a "Living Life on the Veg" lifestyle can be an exciting new opportunity for you to look and feel better, too!

LET'S FIRST LOOK AT WHAT HAPPENS WHEN WE AREN'T "LIVING LIFE ON THE VEG"

Many of us are overfed with quantities of food and yet undernourished. We eat too many calories, yet they are what we call empty—lacking necessary nutrients. Resultantly, we remain hungry, because the foods (food products) we are eating are not nurturing our body because they are nutrient deficient. Calories are not the biggest issue; think about 250 calories in a candy bar, versus 250 calories in fruits. It is the TYPE and quality of the food source of the calorie that matters. Fats, carbohydrates and proteins are all metabolized differently. Instead of eating foods that sustain and support us in our everyday lives, we eat a lot of processed foods and those that satisfy cravings for salt, fat, and sweets. Don't feel bad. We have all been set up by the food industry—especially by the corporations that own the fast-food places we see in our cities and towns—to *want* these foods. As a result, kids grow up wanting a salty, fatty, sugary "meal" with a toy as a lure, instead of a healthier option such as an avocado tomato sandwich and a smoothie.

Do you realize that many of the foods you are eating are man-made? Did you know there are food scientists employed by food product companies who study the science of the physiological and psychological reasons we eat, and what makes us want to continue to eat? These food scientists work to create foods that are addictive so we will want to eat more and buy more. They research ways to make *processed* foods "*safe*" for ingesting into our bodies. Doesn't this sound wrong? Doesn't that mean that processed foods are not made by nature and have to be *altered* for us to be *able* to consume them? Could it be that by eating these foods, we have cardiac disease, cancer, and diabetes in the top ten causes of death in the United States?

"WE COMMIT SUICIDE WITH FOOD."

—DR. JOEL FUHRMAN, family physician, author

Dr. David A. Kessler, former commissioner of the Food and Drug Administration (FDA) has written extensively about the hijacking of the American diet by the fast-food industry and was himself once obese. His book *Fast Carbs, Slow Carbs: The Simple Truth About Food, Weight, and Disease* chronicles the damage that our diets can do to us and the planet, and suggests alternatives.

DECEPTIVE LABELING

There are many buzzwords to look out for in the marketing of food that entice us as consumers to buy foods that aren't healthy and are not in our best interest. Words like "low-fat," "natural," "healthy," "lean," "grass-fed," "free range," "pole caught," and "diet" are meant to get your attention as healthy options, but this wording misleads consumers. Companies even use the word "Organic" in their company name so you will think their products are organic. These and other words are frequently used on the labels of products containing unhealthy and unnatural ingredients.

One way to check if a food is healthy is if you can't understand the ingredients on the label, avoid it, or at the very least, research what that ingredient is so you are informed about what is entering your cells, organs, and tissues.

Think about the bright orange color of certain brands or flavors of chips and the neon blue or green color of a sports drink. Where does that artificial dye coloring go once you eat or drink it? The packaging may even say something like "natural flavor," to make us think something from nature is in it, when the "natural flavor" may be an added chemical compound. This is why it is so important to look at the ingredients on the food labels of your foods and drinks.

So-called "food products," which food scientists create, include harmful ingredients such as dyes, preservatives, stabilizers, saturated and other fats, cholesterol, sodium, sugar, GMOs, high fructose corn syrup, hydrogenated oils, artificial flavors, and chemicals. These additives harm us by damaging the endothelium, the delicate and protective lining of the cardiovascular system vasculature. They cause inflammation, oxidization, plaque buildup in our arteries, and constriction throughout the cardiovascular system.

Chemicals and additives such as those found in chips, sodas, processed juices, snacks, cakes, fried foods, and foods made with refined flour and sugar contribute further to the "Cardiac Bermuda Triangle."

Our passport to this destination is stamped every time we buy and eat these foods because taste, convenience, appealing packaging, and clever marketing, branding, and advertising control our consumer decision-making. We are programmed to want to get our passport stamped for the "Cardiac Bermuda Triangle" every time we see a commercial, advertisement, billboard or signage announcing another fast food option.

SAY "NO" TO GMO

In addition to deceptive labeling, a controversial strategy of the food industry is the use of GMOs (Genetically Modified Organism). Currently, most of the corn, soybean, and canola crops in the U.S. have been genetically modified unless they are labeled organic. Food producers are getting around full transparency on food labeling by using a QR code (a square box of dots on the label) to state in a hidden way that they are GMO products. Do you as a customer in a grocery store routinely scan the QR codes on products when you are shopping? Is it right that a farmer should have to pay thousands and thousands of dollars for the USDA Organic certification, as nature originally intended this food, yet GMO is largely free of certification fees to the GMO farmer and GMO content is *hidden* from the consumer, embedded in a QR code?

> To check what the QR code means, open your phone camera app as if you are taking a picture, using the back camera lens to focus on the QR code. If the product or site does not come

up, then you may need an app that reads QR codes. Try it here! What appears? See what information comes up when you scan a QR code on a food product label at the store.

Reflection Questions: Why did a pharmaceutical company purchase a pesticide and GMO crop producing company? Is it so they can create the drugs that "cure" illnesses caused by eating these GMO products? What consumer protection do we have here when the same governing body oversees food and drugs? Isn't the same governing body overseeing pharmaceuticals and the pesticides together, instead of separately?

"THESE YOUNG PEOPLE ARE SAYING WE ALL HAVE A RIGHT TO KNOW WHAT IS IN THE AIR WE BREATHE, IN THE WATER WE DRINK, AND IN THE FOOD WE EAT. IT IS OUR RESPONSIBILITY TO LEAVE THIS PLANET CLEANER AND GREENER. THAT MUST BE OUR LEGACY."

—JOHN LEWIS, American statesman, civil rights leader

GMO crops have genes that have been altered, to an unnatural state, for example, to prevent browning or reduce crop deaths despite extremely heavy pesticide, herbicide, and fungicide use. Some GMO crops have been modified to internally produce their own stew of chemicals, meaning they can't be washed off. Non-GMO verified products do not include genetically modified components, but may still contain various harmful chemicals not permitted in certified organics.

Organic crops are better for us, for farmers, and the planet, are more naturally nutritious, and decrease our exposure to dangerous chemicals. But we are fighting a food industry that is Goliath to our David. The full extent of all the possible risks of consuming genetically altered foods is still unknown. Bees are dying from these chemicals, and we need bees to pollinate our food plants. Instead of banning the use of bee killing chemicals, scientists have created *robotic bees*. Please look this up and research this, so you are informed. It is really shocking.

Isn't there something dreadfully wrong going on here with our food supply and nature? Until long term scientific study is done, avoiding GMO products and their poisons and carcinogens when possible would be safer than ingesting them. In short: there are still many unanswered questions about how modern foods and beverages will affect our bodies.

> **Organic produce labels:** As much as possible, choose produce items labeled with a number starting with "9," which signifies that they are organic.

MINDFULLY MUNCH

Many of us don't think twice about popping chips into our mouths or eating a block of cut up cheese, served with crackers full of inflammatory chemicals and fillers. We thought that the cheese was dairy and therefore good for us. We thought the (gluten) in grains was good for us. We thought a pizza full of cheese (our calcium) and sausage (our protein) was good for us. Most of us don't realize how deeply connected our food intake and emotions are until something is omitted. We may feel like we lose freedom and happiness, or betray our traditions and culture when we leave certain things off the menu, however, the good news is that we can make new traditions that fuel our bodies in different and better ways.

At first, cutting out excessive sugar, salt and foods that are "fun," seems like you are losing a lot, but what you gain (health, vitality and reversal of disease processes) is priceless. You cannot *buy* your health, but you can *invest* in it with healthy foods. Just as you learned to eat the foods that are bad for your health, it is possible to learn *not* to eat them, and to enjoy healthy foods instead.

> You may even adopt your own personal food culture mindset from one of: **"I want that, but I cannot have it."**
>
> To a mindset of: **"I can have it, but I don't want it."**
>
> (Because now you know better!)

"AN OUNCE OF PREVENTION IS WORTH A POUND OF CURE."
—**BENJAMIN FRANKLIN**, politician, founding father, civic activist

---

It helps to remember that our body is constantly at work to help us. All we need to do is give ourselves the nutrition, rest and support it needs so it can do its job in keeping us healthy and in the balance of homeostasis. That's all it wants from you. Every time we put something into our body that is damaging, it moves us into a state of "dis-ease" or "disease." The body has been interrupted in homeostasis. Eventually, if you continue that behavior, the body cannot fight disease anymore. As a result, we get illnesses like cardiac disease, cancers, obesity, diabetes and may other ailments. Wouldn't it be better to work together with our body? We can, by moving to plant-based nutrition.

THE POWER OF PLANTS

The Whole Food Plant Based (WFPB) credo involves also changing our thoughts from a "diet" mentality—which has such a negative connotation of lack and punishment—to a nutrition mentality: We are *nurturing* our body with our food.

"LET FOOD BE THY MEDICINE AND MEDICINE BE THY FOOD."
—HIPPOCRATES, "The Father of Medicine"

When whole plant foods—foods as close to their natural state as possible—are used to heal and nourish the body, we have control over our health and quality of life. Plants, together with their phytonutrients, antioxidants, plant protein, plant sterols, enzymes, and fiber, offer our body health through their teamwork with our body processes. Diseases of the heart, cancers, diabetes, and other illnesses, can often be prevented through nutrition and lifestyle. Those following a plant-based nutrition lifestyle also have a reduced exposure to toxins, drugs hormones and chemicals found in animal products. Isn't this sounding even better, now?

How do we support our heart health to avoid getting a stamp to the "Cardiac Bermuda Triangle" on our passport? Well, we don't get on the airplane that is going there. The good news is that you can even erase the stamps on your passport if you have taken trips there. In his book, *UnDo It! How Simple Lifestyle Changes Can Reverse Most Chronic Diseases*, world-renowned cardiologist Dr. Dean Ornish shares that through his years of scientific studies, he has proven that we can reverse and prevent cardiac and other diseases by four key principles:

Eat Well, Move More, Stress Less, and Love More.

This is such great news! In a July 16, 2014, story in the Washington Post, Ornish talks about cheeseburgers and yoga and what they mean for heart health, saying: "I'll show a cartoon of doctors busily mopping up the floor [around] a sink overflowing without also turning off the faucet. And it's a great metaphor—that if you don't turn off the faucet, if you don't treat the underlying cause, even if you mop up the floor, even if you do a bypass graft or put a stent in, you're not changing the underlying condition that led to it and so more often than not, those clog up as well. It's like changing your oil filter without changing your oil: It just clogs up again. Or when people get put on cardiac drugs or cholesterol-lowering drugs or statins, things like that: What are they generally told, when the patient says, "How long do I have to take this?" And what does the doctor say? "Forever," right? How long do I have to mop the floor? Forever. Well, why don't I just turn off the faucet?"

Many people, like "Mr. Ain't Happening" want to hear that the answer is to take a quick pill like a statin with their fast food burger to offset or decrease illness. The disease process, the bad foods they eat, still keeps the faucet running and the cause of disease is still there, no matter how much mopping you do. The answer is to turn off the faucet by switching to healthy foods like fruits and vegetables, and adopt healthy lifestyle choices. Then, you won't have to mop up the floor and unnecessarily struggle for good health.

> You gain better health when you give up things that are bad for you.

The road to health is an ongoing journey, and the food choices we make can lead us down two different health paths, either toward wellness or toward illness. Which path you go on is based on your daily decisions.

Reflection Questions: Think about what you ate so far today. Did these foods help your body? How do you feel? Did you enjoy preparing what you ate? Did you eat because you were hungry? Do you enjoy the taste and savor the food? What improvements can you make? You can use the back of your journal pages to record what you eat each day. This is a very interesting exercise to see how many toxins we exposed our body to and how many nourishing things we gave our body.

GIVING THANKS

Take a thoughtful time-out the next time you eat. Look at the food and take a moment to be thankful for it, for all the people involved in bringing it to your plate, for the plant using the sunshine to grow itself, for the nourishment it will bring to your cells and heart and all the organs of your body and your soul. Give thanks because this food will nurture you and in your moment of gratitude, it will bring you joy.

Whole Food Plant Based (WFPB) nutrition means eating the whole plant as much as possible; foods such as fruits, vegetables, leafy greens, legumes, beans, whole grains and a handful of nuts and seeds. What does this look like in a meal? It means instead of a burger on a bleached white flour bun with preservatives, hormones, antibiotics, pesticides and GMO, accompanied by cheese, bacon, fries, and a soda, we are enjoying an organic sautéed garlic, spinach, bean and rice burrito, nutritional yeast instead of grated cheese, with tomato mango salsa we made ourselves on a sprouted whole grain tortilla, washed down with a hot green tea. From what you have learned so far, how might the first meal above be harmful for the body and the vegan meal be healing for the body?

One thing you won't miss about giving up meat: the most difficult parts of cooking it; the hazards of touching raw meat, cross-contamination of diseases from animal products, de-boning, trimming animal fat, and cooking the meat sufficiently so we don't get sick.

In contrast, plants are easy. Plants have no blood, feathers, organs, bones, skin or diseases to contend with. Prepping plants take far less time and effort than prepping meat. With a little patience, creativity, and open-mindedness, the possibilities of plant-based dishes are truly amazing.

"SO... WHERE DO YOU GET YOUR PROTEIN?"

This is the most frequent question asked by non-vegans when considering going vegan. Well, where do the cows get their protein from? You guessed it—plants. Most protein found in animal products originally came from plants, like when a cow eats grass. Getting our protein straight from plants cuts out the middleman, the animals.

> All protein needs can be met with plants.

It is hard to become protein deficient while consuming an adequate amount of calories, with a variety of plant products. Protein is in almost everything, even fruit. Protein is essential for building and repairing tissues, but it is often overconsumed. We don't need to spend more money to add expensive protein powders to our smoothies when nature has already provided what we need. Athletes do not need to increase their protein intake. I recommend watching the movie *The Game Changers*, found online, about how athletes can thrive on plant-based nutrition. For more information about the overconsumption of protein, please see the book *Protein Aholic: How Our Obsession with Meat is Killing Us and What We Can Do About It*, by Garth Davis, MD.

It is best to enjoy our foods as close to their natural form as possible, with nothing healthy removed and nothing unhealthy added. The closer foods are to their natural form—what we call whole foods, the more they may benefit our health. Selecting local, seasonal, and organic foods when possible promotes healthy and planet-friendly consumption of our resources and, when in season, is less costly.

Eating whole foods can also lessen your risk of disease and even reverse those conditions you have. If you are taking unhealthy foods and fat from meat off of your plate, your Type 2 diabetes should improve because by decreasing meat intake, you have fired "Fat," the bouncer!

> It is important to note that if you are diabetic and taking insulin, you will need to monitor your blood sugars closely as you transition to fewer animal products while adding more fresh fruits and vegetables.
>
> There is a chart in the back of your book to record your morning glucose daily. You will need to share your change in your nutrition and your blood glucose records with your doctor, who may put you on a different administration plan for glucose control, as your blood sugar may naturally go down.

Remember, don't blame the banana or the potato for high blood sugar, blame it on the bouncer, "Fat," who doesn't allow those healthy sources of energy into the cell.

> **PRO TIP**: When deciding if something is healthy, consider your other options. For example, if you are going to dinner, a mock meat (man-made alternatives to meat burgers) burger may be a healthier choice than an animal-based burger, but it is definitely less healthy than a WFPB (Whole Food Plant Based) veggie bean burger. Once you have this awareness, it is easy to determine healthy choices when dining in or eating out.

> **PRO TIP**: In a pinch, it is possible to make a meal entirely out of vegetable side dishes in a restaurant. Restaurants have become more accommodating for vegans, and if you ask, most will happily provide options for you. You can even call the restaurant ahead to see what vegan accommodations they offer.

> **PRO TIP**: If someone is having a BBQ, bring your own veggie burgers and veggies for the grill. Who knows—by your newfound health and vitality, you may be introducing someone else to a new healthy lifestyle by your example.

PRO TIP: What if you are alone in a house full of meat eaters? How can you make win-win meals for all? Can you include a protein based "main dish" such as quinoa, or rice and beans, without yourself having the actual meat? Can you make extra sides of vegetables to enjoy? Can you slip "Meatless Mondays" into the weekly meal planning? How can this be resolved to be a win-win meal for everyone, while at the same time striving for healthier options? Can we move from less healthy meat options to those having less fat, like from bacon to turkey bacon and then to a plant-based bacon?

HOW DO YOU START A PLANT-BASED DIET?

Here are some steps to get you on your way to plant-based eating:

CLEAN OUT THE KITCHEN

Get rid of the products that aren't serving your health. Discard processed foods and anything with ingredients you cannot pronounce, or has chemicals, dyes, or preservatives. Look at the way things are marketed and packaged. Do they say "natural" when really, they are not?

GET CREATIVE

Search online for your favorite dishes with the word "vegan." I searched around and found a great recipe for cauliflower "mac-n-cheese" without the pasta or the cheese; just cauliflower. I didn't even miss the pasta, or the cheese! (Fact!)

Websites such as www.milliondollarvegan.com, www.plant poweredkitchen.com, www.cookingwithplants.com, and www.the vegan8.com are fantastic resources for vegan recipes. As you search around, you will find your own favorites. I have listed some amazing cookbooks and websites for your plant-based food journey in the "Resource Boutique" at the end of your book.

EXPERIMENT WITH SPICES

Try different ways of changing your recipe flavors by adding in spices to your taste. Pick whatever you are drawn to and feel would add that little extra pow! to the taste. Have fun and get creative. Go completely off-recipe and add in your own spices to taste to put your signature on the dish.

GET ORGANIZED

When shopping for a recipe, organize a list of ingredients from the same department in the grocery store to make it easier to shop.

PRO TIP: Shop with a full belly! You are bound to have more things "jump into your cart" if you grocery shop when you are hungry than if you shop with something in your stomach. Have your ongoing grocery list at the ready so you won't forget items needed for a food creation you are planning.

SEEK AND SHOP FOR VARIETY IN THE FOODS YOU EAT FROM DAY TO DAY

Rotate what you eat daily to get better maximum vitamin use by your body from your foods. Purchase fruits and vegetables that are in season, which will be less expensive, because they are plentiful.

STOCK YOUR PANTRY WITH SHELF-STABLE PRODUCTS

As much as possible, stock your panty with and cook with gluten-free healthier options such as brown rice, basmati rice, black rice, red rice, wild rice, jasmine rice, teff, amaranth, gluten free oats, quinoa, millet, sorghum and buckwheat. Keep a variety of other shelf-stable staples on hand, such as dried beans, peas, pasta, canned goods that are BPA-free, pasta sauces and any other basics for your plant-based kitchen.

ENJOY 1-2 SERVINGS OF GRAINS DAILY

GO GLUTEN-FREE

As much as possible, avoid gluten products such as wheat, spelt, kamut, farro, durum, bulgur, semolina, barley, rye, tricale, and oats containing gluten. For great information and resources about gluten and its role in health, see: www.wholegrainscouncil.org

> **PRO TIP:** Dried pastas are made from a variety of ingredients, not just semolina or wheat or other gluten-containing ingredients. There are high protein pasta options to try, such as lentil, quinoa, chickpea, and edamame.

> **PRO TIP:** Stay saucy! I find that pasta noodles are best when cooked fresh per meal, as opposed to cooking the pasta and using it combined with sauce as a leftover. Instead, make lots of sauce and cook your pasta fresh to go with the leftover sauce.

ENJOY LEGUMES

Beans are a great source of fiber, and they feed our gut bacteria, which in turn helps improve our immunity. Opt for dried peas, beans and lentils or canned, low-sodium options. Varieties to try: pigeon peas, green peas, split peas, pinto beans, kidney beans, lima beans, butter beans, kidney beans, black beans, pink beans, navy beans, adzuki beans, fava beans, edamame beans, cannellini beans, garbanzo beans, great northern beans, broad beans, mung beans, green beans, yard-long beans, green lentils, brown lentils, red lentils, gold lentils, black lentils, and more. As you can see, there are many options to use and to substitute for other kinds in your recipes.

HAVE CANNED AND JARRED STAPLES ON HAND

Keep some jarred salsas, tomato sauces, vinegars, and coconut aminos as your back-ups to have on hand. Coconut aminos are a delicious, lower sodium (high B12) replacement for soy sauce and can be used in place of a balsamic vinegar in a salad dressing, or sprinkled directly on your veggies to brighten their taste. Dates, agave and maple syrup are excellent options for adding sweetness to many recipes.

GET PROPER KITCHEN TOOLS

It is worth the investment and makes your cooking organization much easier. Below is a list of kitchen tools I recommend:

- Stainless Steel Saucepan
- Large Stainless Steel Pot
- Colander
- Roasting pan
- Baking Sheets
- Citrus Juicer
- Grater
- Blender (preferably high speed)
- Food Processor
- Spatula
- Wooden Spoon
- Measuring Cups
- Measuring Spoons
- Pyrex Baking Dish
- Toaster Oven

- Vegetable Steamer
- Coffee Press or single use pour over coffee maker with #2 size non-dyed paper filters
- Glass Jars and Storage Containers
- Large and Small Cast Iron Skillets

> **PRO TIP:** Get rid of toxic Teflon-coated cookware and aluminum cookware. Use stainless steel and cast iron cookware instead. As much as possible, use glass containers versus plastic. Avoid heating food in plastic in the microwave, due to the potential for leaching the plastic into the food.

> **PRO TIP:** Tomatoes have a reaction with the iron of a cast iron skillet, so do not cook tomatoes in the cast iron, use stainless steel instead. Season the cast iron regularly. Look up how to season and care for cast iron. It should not be washed with soap and water as it could rust and requires special care.

OTHER KITCHEN NECESSITIES:
- **Sharp Knives.** Purchase a small paring knife, large chef knife and a medium serrated knife.
- **Cutting board.** Wooden cutting boards are ideal, as we want to eliminate plastic from our life as much as possible.

> **PRO TIP**: Place a wet paper towel under the cutting board to prevent it from moving or sliding as you cut on it. To eliminate warping, wash and dry it, and store flat immediately after use.

As you finesse your chef skills, you may want to incorporate these items:

- Wok
- Mixer
- Air Fryer
- Spiralizer
- Crock Pot
- Coffee Percolator
- Small Coffee Grinder

> **PRO TIP**: Crock pots are great because you can "set it and forget it." Crock pots slow cook the food, and are a perfect way to make a veggie stew or meat-free chili or soup on a cold winter day. I make sure I will be home all day to attend to an electrical appliance turned on and in use, plus I get to enjoy the smell of all the seasonings and foods mingling as they cook.

GET SPICED UP

One of the reasons we get hooked on certain foods is because of the flavorings and spices on them, not necessarily the base food under the spices. Buffalo chicken wings can be switched out for vegan Buffalo cauliflower nibbles with the same spices, but with a different, healthier cauliflower base. Plant-based cooking high in fiber, vitamins, minerals, and antioxidants does not have to consist of bland and boring meals. Instead of reliance on harmful additives or large amounts of fat, sugar, and salt, use spices and herbs that can add a lot of flavor, at the same time acting as your "Farm-acy" due to their health benefits. Adding freshly squeezed citrus juices and zests (grating the washed rind of lemon, lime, or orange) can brighten and enhance many recipes. There are a variety of flavor options to choose from or customize your own. Herbs and spices may be fresh or dried. Dried options may be whole or ground. Freshly ground seasonings (such as using a grinder on peppercorns or nutmeg) have a more intense flavor than pre-ground ones.

Examples of the many spices to play with in your recipes are: anise, nutmeg, chipotle, curry, marjoram, coriander, chive, parsley, cilantro, thyme, cayenne, red pepper flakes, cinnamon, clove, cardamom, bay leaf, turmeric, pepper, Himalayan salt, cumin, oregano, smoked paprika, rosemary, sage, basil, dill, fennel, mint, black pepper, lemon pepper, cayenne pepper, white pepper, and chili powder for starters.

PRO TIP: Do you have a windowsill where you might be able to grow pots of your own rosemary, oregano, mint, basil, and chives? These are

my "favorite five" herbs I find I most frequently use. It is really rewarding to nourish a plant that you potted or even purchased already in a
pot, knowing it provides you with health benefits reciprocally.

Now that you have information about the fundamentals and the
supplies to optimize your kitchen cooking experience, let's decode
food labels, which contain nutritional information.

THE BASICS OF THE NUTRITION FACTS LABEL

The food label will tell you how many servings a food item has per
container. You may be surprised to know that you may have been
consuming 2-3 serving-sized portions. No judgments here! I've been
there, too! The nutrition label will also give you the recommended
daily nutritional allowance provided per serving. This is the funda-
mental start to learning about your nutritional journey with food.

The Physicians Committee for Responsible Medicine (www.pcrm.
org) has some wonderful tools on their website to help to read a
food label, and to get you started on your vegan journey. A tip from
PCRM: start from the top and work your way to the bottom.

MONITOR PORTION/SERVING SIZE

What is the serving size? Are you consuming 2-3 times the serving
size? If so, you will need to double or triple the nutritional information along with those extra portions. How many calories are there?
For example, if you have a three-serving portion size, you will be
tripling the amount of calories, saturated fat, salt, sugar, and other

items as well. Are you considering the recommended daily allowance (RDA) nutritional energy intake plan of 2,000 calories a day for women and 2,500 calories a day for men? Those sneaky calories in packaged foods can add up quickly, so be mindful of your portions.

MAKE THE CALORIES COUNT

How many calories are there per serving? Do those calories contain a lot of inflammatory sugar? It is important to note that it is common when switching to a whole-food, plant-based diet to not be eating *enough* calories. Really? Yes, that's right. Plant foods generally have a lower *density* of calories, and a higher water and fiber content than animal products and processed foods. Those looking to lose weight will achieve optimum results by consuming more water-dense vegetables such as cucumbers than starchy foods such as potatoes and grains.

Make sure you are eating enough. Consider the "fill factor" in the calories when consuming a half pound burger with bacon and cheese on it, plus chili fries and a milkshake, versus a vegan burrito and an iced tea. You have space for some veggies on the side or some fruit or a nice side salad.

MONITOR THE FAT CONTENT

What is the total fat, and is it the unwanted kind of saturated or trans-fat? The goal: 2-3 grams of fat per serving. Remember Fat, the bouncer at the club? Fat keeps insulin from doing the good work to bring glucose into the cell for energy. Fat contributes to the progression of diabetes. We want to keep our fat intake low. Note: do not be fooled by foods labeled as "low fat." Remember the food scientists at work in their lab to alter food products for your body. A package of food may be labeled low fat, yet so is an orange. A certain famous sandwich cookie can be labeled vegan, but it is a nutritional mess. By weight, an ounce of olive oil has a lot more calories than an ounce of fruit or vegetables. Minimize oils in your diet; they are highly caloric and can contribute to vascular disease.

> **PRO TIP**: Use (organic) coconut oil as a cooling skin moisturizer. Do not eat it or cook with it!

> **PRO TIP**: Instead of cooking with oils, you can try other ways to prepare foods such as steaming, or sautéing foods in a bit of vegetable broth. Vegetable broth can usually be found in the organic section or the soup section of your supermarket. You can try making your own by resourcing recipes online.

> **PRO TIP**: For healthier fats with protein, eat nut and seed butters (in moderation), but pour off the extra oil floating on top when you open a jar of nut butter to save on calories and fat consumption.

IS THERE CHOLESTEROL AND HOW MUCH?

The label ideally has zero cholesterol. If you aren't eating anything with animal products in it, you will not be taking in excess artery-blocking cholesterol.

MONITOR SODIUM

We want to keep our sodium (salt) intake low. Eating a lot of foods with sodium can increase our blood pressure, creating a strain on the heart and other organs, too. Daily sodium intake per the RDA is less than 2,300 mg.

> PRO TIP: Try using sea kelp seasoning for flavor, or other herbal seasonings, instead of salt. Keep looking at those nutrition labels on your food, because salt (sodium) really adds up quickly. Notice if you are reaching for the salt shaker before you even taste your food.

CHECK THE CARBOHYDRATES

Carbohydrates are a combination of fibers, sugars and starch. When you read the label, you will only see fiber and sugar broken out. The balance is starch. There is a lot of information about types of carbohydrates online if you would like to research this further.

LOOK FOR FOODS WITH FIBER

Although protein is definitely important, the question that is equally as important is: "Where do you get your fiber?" The benefits of fiber consumption are especially helpful for those seeking cardiovascular health improvements. Increased fiber intake has been shown to reduce the risk of heart disease, diabetes, certain cancers, obesity, and of course, constipation. Reduction in cardiovascular disease risks have been achieved by simply having an additional seven grams of fiber daily. Fiber feeds the good bacteria in the gut, and helps control cholesterol, blood sugar, and blood pressure. Fiber also reduces the transit time it takes for food to get through the gut, helping the body clear out waste, including the removal of excess cholesterol. What is not to like about our new friend, fiber?

Fiber can be found in many delicious plants such as jackfruit, lentils, beans, broccoli, greens, sweet potatoes, potatoes, chia seeds, peas, raspberries, dates, prunes, pears, apples, and (preferably gluten-free) more nutritious whole grains.

> **PRO TIP**: Do not strain or push when you are making poops, as this also puts strain on your heart! Before reaching for a laxative, try incorporating fibrous prunes and dates into your nutrition. They make a great filling snack that will "get you moving."

MINIMIZE SUGAR AND SWEETENERS

Avoid sugar and especially high fructose corn syrup. This sugary sweetener is mostly made from GMO corn, and is an inflammatory sugar. As much as possible, be thoughtful about your sugar intake. Avoid sugars and make it a treat with benefits, when you do have it. For a thoughtfully chosen dessert with health benefits, select a square of dark chocolate. According to the Harvard School of Public Health, the health benefits of dark chocolate are its flavonols, which help the blood vessels to increase nitric oxide, which lowers blood pressure. Why not enjoy a few fibrous dates and a brazil nut with your piece of dark chocolate for a tasty desert filled with health benefits?

Artificial sweeteners are just that: an artificial product meant to trick your body into thinking you are having a sweet. Recall those food scientists busily crafting food products.

PRO TIP: Look at the nutrition label of what you are eating or drinking. How much sugar is in your food? Take a look at the neon coloring of a sports drink. Is this natural for your body to absorb? What are the ingredients on the label? How many grams of sugar are in it per serving?

4.2 grams of sugar = 1 teaspoon of sugar = 16 calories

The 34 grams of sugar in one single-serving bottle of a sports drink I looked at had the equivalent of 8 teaspoons of sugar. If you drank this, you would be consuming the equivalent of eating 8 teaspoons of sugar. This is not including the rest of the sugar (and calories) you have had in your foods that day. Let's say you are an athlete, and during your game, you drank two of these sugar filled sports drinks, the equivalent of 16 teaspoons of sugar. Imagine spooning that sugar into your mouth. Afterwards, you are off to the diner to celebrate the big win! If you have a soda with a bacon cheeseburger and fries, and then ice cream on the way home, how does this one day of eating stack up in fostering obesity, diabetes, heart disease, cancer and inflammation? This one afternoon of sugar deserves *two* passport entry stamps for a trip to the "Cardiac Bermuda Triangle." You might have a thin body, being athletic, but your arteries could be clogged, and your cells could be filling with this fat, too, leading to diabetes. Remember, we cannot see heart disease or diabetes on the outside of a person.

From the example above, it is easy to see why heart disease, obesity, and diabetes are so rampant in our society, and yet they are mostly preventable when we eat for health.

CHECK FOR EXCESS PROTEIN

Per the PCRM, 10–20% of our daily calories should be found in protein. Did you know fruits contain about 5% protein? Vegetables up to 15%? Grains, 10–15%? Beans 20–50%? The good news for you to hear is that we are not in danger of being protein deficient if we are eating a wide variety and enough of these foods.

Whole food plant-based protein sources are easily found in tofu (soybean), tempeh (fermented soybeans), lentils, green peas, legumes, pumpkin and hemp seeds, whole grains, spinach, broccoli, kale and more. Mock meats have plant extracted protein, but tend to be processed (created by food scientists) and are high in sodium and fat. On the plus side, mock meats lack cholesterol, choline, hormones and animal fat, unlike animal-based burgers. They are great to enjoy as you transition from animal meat to healthier food options.

Enjoy 2-3 servings a day of legumes, beans, tofu and lentils. Enjoy 1-2 servings of raw, unsalted nuts and seeds (a small handful) per day.

Visit **www.fda.gov** for current information regarding the RDA

(Recommended Daily Allowance) of fat, carbs, sodium, fiber, protein, and calories you should be consuming on a daily basis.

In addition to the FDA information, read the *ingredients* on the food label. Are there additives, preservatives, GMOs, food dyes, chemicals, or things you cannot pronounce in this product? Be a label detective, selecting food options that help your body in its quest for ongoing homeostasis.

Note: Newer food labels will reflect vitamins and minerals that we may be deficient in, such as vitamin D, Calcium, Iron, and Potassium.

VITAMIN B12

It is important to have reliable sources of vitamin B12 daily. It is an essential vitamin that our bodies do not make. The recommended daily allowance is 2.4 micrograms. B12 is important, especially if you are vegan. Crucial for red blood cell formation, DNA synthesis, and normal nerve function, vitamin B12 is an essential vitamin. Animal products are sources of B12, but they are also sources of cholesterol, saturated fat, hormones and antibiotics that we do not want in our body. It is a common misconception that B12 can only be sourced from animal products.

Animals raised for food are almost always supplemented with B12. Neither animals nor plants make vitamin B12. Instead, tiny microbes blanketing the planet via our soil are responsible for its creation. In the modern sanitized world, with chlorinated drinking water, loss of viable topsoil and extra thorough produce washing, a reliable source of vitamin B12 is needed. vitamin B12 is abundantly found in foods such as nutritional yeast, duckweed, nori, (dried seaweed) spirulina, chlorella, fortified cereals, and plant milks. Nutritional yeast is a tasty addition to the plant-based kitchen and an excellent source of B12. Nutritional yeast lends an incredibly cheesy flavor when sprinkled on potatoes, pasta, veggies, and whole grains, or when added to just about anything savory. It is even better with a little garlic and onion powder for added flavor. Nutritional yeast is a really close taste substitute for grated parmesan cheese. Try it the next time you make pasta. You can also take a B Complex vitamin supplement to ensure you are getting your B12 as well as other B vitamins.

PRO TIP: For other options for more B12, use tamari, or liquid aminos (which tastes like a balsamic vinegar), as a salad dressing with a sprinkle of olive oil. There is even a coconut-based version of aminos. There are low sodium options as well.

CALCIUM

Calcium is necessary for our bone growth and for many cell functions. Calcium can be found in beans and lentils, sesame seeds, broccoli, bok choy, kale, collard greens, edamame, tofu, figs, oatmeal, fortified cereals, chia seeds, and oranges.

Dairy is not necessary to obtain calcium. Animal-based products such as milks, cheeses, ice creams, sour creams, yogurts and products made using milk, such as milk chocolate, include the same toxins, drugs, chemicals, cholesterol, and animal fats that meats have.

Drinking just one cup of milk per day has been associated with an increased risk of breast cancer. It has also been concluded that dairy may increase the risk of bone fractures, along with endometrial and prostate cancer. We now know that we have plenty of vegan (non-dairy) options for these same products.

OMEGA 3

One to two tablespoons of flax seeds, chia seeds, or walnuts may be consumed daily for Omega 3, important for anti-inflammation. They can be used in many recipes, smoothies, and as toppings for salads or non-dairy desserts. Flax and chia seeds can even be used to replace eggs.

PRO TIP: To make one flax or chia "egg," use one tablespoon of ground chia seed or flaxseed mixed with three tablespoons of water. Stir frequently. After the mixture thickens for about 15 minutes, the "egg" can be added to your recipe. There are many options that you can use as a substitute for eggs as a binder in your recipes, such as applesauce or even beans.

Enjoy 2 tablespoons of ground chia or ground flax per day.

SELENIUM

Selenium is an antioxidant that may also protect against heart disease and inflammation. Just 1–3 Brazil nuts a day will reach daily selenium intake needs. But Brazil nuts are not just for selenium. They are also good sources of vitamin E, copper, manganese, phosphorus, and magnesium. They can be stuffed inside dates, eaten with dark chocolate, put in smoothies, or chopped and added onto salads. Other sources of selenium are green or brown lentils and pecans; but Brazil nuts are the highest by far.

IRON

You too can be as strong as Popeye was after he ate his can of spinach. It is a common misconception that animal products are needed for iron. Dark green vegetables, leafy greens, beans, nuts and seeds, dried fruit, whole grains, and black strap molasses are great sources of iron. Cooking with cast iron cookware can leach minute amounts of iron into your food, giving you an added benefit of iron. Combining a citrus with a leafy green can increase the amount of iron your body absorbs. Increase your iron intake by squeezing lemon on top of sautéed spinach or incorporating lemon into the salad dressing for a spinach or other leafy green salad.

Supplements: It is very important to check with your doctor before supplementing because there could be interactions between the vitamins or supplements and your medications, and you also may need a test to get your base level of certain vitamins.

Based on your lab results, speak with your doctor about supplementing any of the following vitamins you may be deficient in: Zinc, vitamin A, C, E, Selenium, D, B2, B6, B12, Folic Acid, and Co-Q10.

VITAMIN D

Vitamin D is especially important in the winter months and in colder environments where you may not be able to get the sun exposure the warmer climates do. Have your blood levels checked and speak with your doctor about supplementation, if needed. Vitamin D, actually a hormone, is critical for helping our immune system work optimally.

CO-Q10

Speak to your doctor about supplementing with Co-Q10, especially if you are on a statin.

BERGAMOT

Speak with your doctor about taking this to see if it may help nudge your cholesterol levels down.

> PRO TIP: If you are taking vitamins or supplements, take them with food to avoid nausea, unless otherwise instructed.

WATER

Water is very important for your organs and tissues to work optimally. If you drink caffeinated drinks such as coffee or tea, ensure you are also hydrating to replace the diuretic effect of the caffeine. Diuretics make us eliminate more urine, which can make us dehydrated. A good rule is to have a glass of water for every cup of coffee or caffeinated beverage.

Opt for water and teas, such as green tea or herbal teas, instead of milk, sugary drinks, diet beverages, and sodas. Commercial juices and bottled teas are loaded with chemicals such as aspartame, and similar falsely "beneficial" drinks should be avoided. Instead, add washed citrus slices, chunks of peeled cucumber, or frozen fruit to water, adding in health benefits along with their great flavors. Smoothies are preferred over juicing. Even the best and most expensive juicers remove the precious (and beneficial) fiber of the vegetables and fruits. Juicing may also give you a spike in blood glucose levels due to a more rapid gut absorption from the loss of fiber.

> **PRO TIP**: Blending whole fruits and vegetables into a smoothie is a healthy and easy way to get more servings of fruits and veggies daily.

> **PRO TIP**: If you do have a juice or smoothie, rinse your mouth if you cannot brush your teeth immediately afterwards, to prevent cavities. It is a good practice to rinse your mouth out with water after you eat.

WEEKLY HOMEWORK
(CHECK OFF WHEN COMPLETED)

☐ Watch the movie *The Game Changers* (2018) online.

☐ See how creative you can be for a day eating plant-based. Look up recipes for your favorite food but substitute the word vegan instead of a meat. Example: vegan burritos, vegan chili, vegan stew, vegan nachos. Give it a try. Take a picture of your creation and tag @hearttosoulcw on Instagram so I can share it to inspire others.

Day 36: **YOUR HEART TO SOUL DAILY JOURNAL**

DATE: _____

DAILY WEIGHT: _____ **A.M. GLUCOSE:** _____

TODAY'S OVERALL FEELING OF WELLNESS:

1   2   3   4   5   6   7   8   9   10

INTENTION WORD FOR THE DAY: _____

TODAY I ACCOMPLISHED:

☐ Mindful breath work

☐ Mindful meditation (Duration _____)

☐ Joy & Meaning self-care activity: _____

3 THINGS I AM GRATEFUL FOR TODAY:

1.

2.

3.

WHAT'S ON YOUR MIND?

Day 37: YOUR HEART TO SOUL DAILY JOURNAL

DATE: _____

DAILY WEIGHT: _____ A.M. GLUCOSE: _____

TODAY'S OVERALL FEELING OF WELLNESS:

1   2   3   4   5   6   7   8   9   10

INTENTION WORD FOR THE DAY: _____

TODAY I ACCOMPLISHED:

- ☐ Mindful breath work
- ☐ Mindful meditation (Duration _____)
- ☐ Joy & Meaning self-care activity: _____

3 THINGS I AM GRATEFUL FOR TODAY:

1.

2.

3.

WHAT'S ON YOUR MIND?

Day 38: YOUR HEART TO SOUL DAILY JOURNAL

DATE: _____

DAILY WEIGHT:_____   A.M. GLUCOSE:_____

TODAY'S OVERALL FEELING OF WELLNESS:

1   2   3   4   5   6   7   8   9   10

INTENTION WORD FOR THE DAY:_____

TODAY I ACCOMPLISHED:

☐ Mindful breath work

☐ Mindful meditation (Duration _____)

☐ Joy & Meaning self-care activity:_____

3 THINGS I AM GRATEFUL FOR TODAY:

1.

2.

3.

WHAT'S ON YOUR MIND?

Day 39: YOUR HEART TO SOUL DAILY JOURNAL

DATE: _____

DAILY WEIGHT:_____   A.M. GLUCOSE:_____

TODAY'S OVERALL FEELING OF WELLNESS:

1   2   3   4   5   6   7   8   9   10

INTENTION WORD FOR THE DAY:_____

TODAY I ACCOMPLISHED:

☐ Mindful breath work

☐ Mindful meditation (Duration _____)

☐ Joy & Meaning self-care activity:_____

3 THINGS I AM GRATEFUL FOR TODAY:

1.

2.

3.

WHAT'S ON YOUR MIND?

Day 40: YOUR HEART TO SOUL DAILY JOURNAL

DATE: _____

DAILY WEIGHT: _____   **A.M. GLUCOSE:** _____

TODAY'S OVERALL FEELING OF WELLNESS:

1   2   3   4   5   6   7   8   9   10

INTENTION WORD FOR THE DAY: _____

TODAY I ACCOMPLISHED:

☐ Mindful breath work

☐ Mindful meditation (Duration _____)

☐ Joy & Meaning self-care activity: _____

3 THINGS I AM GRATEFUL FOR TODAY:

1.

2.

3.

WHAT'S ON YOUR MIND?

Day 41: **YOUR HEART TO SOUL DAILY JOURNAL**

DATE: _____

DAILY WEIGHT: _____ **A.M. GLUCOSE:** _____

TODAY'S OVERALL FEELING OF WELLNESS:

1   2   3   4   5   6   7   8   9   10

INTENTION WORD FOR THE DAY: _____

TODAY I ACCOMPLISHED:

☐ Mindful breath work

☐ Mindful meditation (Duration _____)

☐ Joy & Meaning self-care activity: _____

3 THINGS I AM GRATEFUL FOR TODAY:

1.

2.

3.

WHAT'S ON YOUR MIND?

Day 42: YOUR HEART TO SOUL DAILY JOURNAL

DATE: _____

DAILY WEIGHT:_____   A.M. GLUCOSE:_____

TODAY'S OVERALL FEELING OF WELLNESS:

1   2   3   4   5   6   7   8   9   10

INTENTION WORD FOR THE DAY:_____

TODAY I ACCOMPLISHED:

☐ Mindful breath work

☐ Mindful meditation (Duration _____)

☐ Joy & Meaning self-care activity:_____

3 THINGS I AM GRATEFUL FOR TODAY:

1.

2.

3.

WHAT'S ON YOUR MIND?

Week 7:

LET YOUR REFRIGERATOR BE YOUR MEDICINE CABINET

You have everything you need already to kick off your new, healthy plan for nutrition. Your "culinary medicine" is as close as your kitchen. Below you will find some ideas about how to stock your "new" medicine cabinet: your refrigerator.

PRODUCE

If possible, purchase fresh produce when it is in season, which means lower, more affordable prices while supply is plentiful. When you can, purchase fresh versus frozen. Frozen produce does have a few benefits to note: frozen fruits and vegetables have almost as many nutrients as fresh produce. Fruits and veggies from the frozen foods section have a much longer shelf life than their fresh counterparts. Frozen items also usually require less prep work because they are pre-cut and washed. Try to select organic produce, even in the freezer section, if possible.

> **PRO TIP:** Frozen fruit is great to have on hand for smoothies. You can avoid discarding over-ripe bananas, for example. Cut them in pieces and freeze them for use in smoothies.

LEAFY GREENS

Nitrates absorbed from the soil into leafy greens are converted to nitrites in the mouth, which naturally decreases blood pressure. Examples of foods containing nitrates are arugula, lettuces, beets, kale, bok choy, cabbage, fennel, and spinach. Think of nitroglycerine tablets used under the tongue in an emergency for opening the blood vessels to relieve chest pain. We have nitrates available in our food that our bodies convert to blood pressure lowering nitrites in nature. How cool is that? This is another great example of how our body uses our food for health homeostasis.

Other great leafy greens to sample are watercress, turnip greens, beet greens, mustard greens, collards, chard, leeks, dandelion greens, seaweed, parsley, green onions, and chives.

> **LEAFY GREENS ALERT!** If you are on any blood thinners, it is important to check with your doctor regarding the quantity of leafy greens and garlic you will consume in your new healthier meals. Garlic and leafy greens may impact the efficacy of blood thinners. Once you get to a consistent state of eating these important foods, your medication can be adjusted to complement this food intake for your optimal blood levels.

Otherwise, if you are not on blood thinning medications, you may enjoy 3 or more servings a day.

STARCHY VEGETABLES

Good, healthy starch can be found in yams, different kinds, colors, and varieties of potatoes such as sweet potatoes, red potatoes, russet potatoes, Yukon potatoes, and fingerling potatoes. Explore different varieties. You will find they have different flavors and consistencies when cooked. Other starches to explore are yucca, taro, corn, carrots, squash varieties such as butternut squash, zucchini squash, spaghetti squash, acorn squash, pumpkin, and parsnips.

NON-STARCHY VEGETABLES

Artichokes, asparagus, beets, onions, broccoli, eggplant, celery, cauliflower, tomatillos, rutabagas, shallots, Brussel sprouts, chayote, cabbage, kohlrabi, bok choy, turnips, radicchio, summer squash, zucchini, radishes, rhubarb, and okra.

Enjoy 3 or more servings a day of starchy or non-starchy vegetables.

AVOCADOS

Let's talk about a big favorite, which is actually a "stone fruit." Avocados deserve their own paragraph. Avocados have a lot of monounsaturated fats in them, which are a "healthy" fat option that helps to increase our "good" cholesterol—the HDL, or high-density lipoprotein cholesterol.

Avocados contain many vitamins, minerals and fiber. Avocados are sources of vitamins C, E, K and B6, riboflavin, niacin, folate, magnesium, and potassium, which our heart enjoys. Avocados are sources of non-inflammatory Omega 3 fatty acids.

> **PRO TIP**: For a do-it-yourself beauty tip to nourish your skin, after washing the outside then scooping out your avocado for your food preparation, you can rub any leftover bits of avocado remaining on the peel on your face or the backs of your hands for a hydrating and soothing mask. Rinse it off before it starts to dry and crack.

> **PRO TIP**: Use washed, organic lemon halves after you have squeezed the lemons to rub on your elbows to both lighten and soften the skin there. Lemon halves can also be placed in the refrigerator on a shelf for a day or two as mini natural "air fresheners." Their washed rinds can be grated to add a "zest" to a dish such as simple pasta with mint and peas and a little garlic.

BERRIES

Berries contain many different antioxidants and vitamins. In his book *Medical Medium: Secrets Behind Chronic and Mystery Illness and How to Finally Heal*, Anthony William discusses the nature of food, and how its growing environment has helped fruit produce vitamins, which lends us those health benefits by eating it.

Berries are a great go-to for breakfast or as a portable snack. Try some of these types of berries with your breakfast: raspberries, goji berries, blueberries, cranberries, blackberries, strawberries, acai, boysenberry, and elderberries.

OTHER FRUITS

Explore and try varieties of cherries, mangos, pears, apples, kiwi, oranges, tangerines, clementines, bananas, grapes, figs, guavas, lychees, kumquats, pomegranate, plums, nectarines, peaches, papayas, pineapples, apricots, persimmons, plantains, passion fruit, pomelo, jackfruit, watermelon, honeydew melons, cantaloupes, lemons, limes, star fruit, dragon fruit, loquats, soursop, and more.

> Enjoy 3 or more servings a day of fruit.

MAKE YOUR KITCHEN A KALEIDOSCOPE

Do you remember playing with kaleidoscopes when you were a kid? Remember how mesmerizing all the colors were? That is how our body feels when we eat a variety of colorful foods; bright, colorful, and in flow with homeostasis.

Colorful fruits and vegetables are well known for being healthy, and they are also a treat for the eyes. Various colors give us clues as to what beneficial treasures are within, such as phytonutrients, (plant nutrients) vitamins and minerals. Edible plants have overlapping nutrients, and they work together in synergy with each other. Variety is very important, because mixing and matching about forty plants a week promotes optimal gut health, and the nutrients can work better together harmoniously for your body. I encourage you to do your own research on all the health benefits of your fruits and vegetables. Here are some of the high points of their colorful superpowers:

RED

Superpower: The carotenoid lycopene. Anti-cancer, anti-oxidant, may protect against heart disease and help blood flow.

Found in: Watermelons, strawberries, beets, tomatoes, red peppers, cherries, cranberries, and grapes.

ORANGE

Superpower: Vitamin C. May improve immune function and fight free radicals.

Found in: Sweet potatoes, pomelo, satsumas, tangerines, oranges, clementines, pumpkin, orange peppers, cantaloupe, papaya, and persimmons.

> **GRAPEFRUIT WARNING:** If you are on *any* medications, avoid grapefruit. It affects the ability of the liver enzymes to properly metabolize your medications, so a drug may become either more toxic or rendered less effective after eating grapefruit.

YELLOW

Superpower: Vitamin A. May improve endothelial function, promote the formation of new cells, and support vision health.

Found in: Yellow peppers, yellow carrots, winter squash, summer squash, spaghetti squash, bananas, and mangoes.

GREEN

Superpower: Vitamin K, nitrates. Aid in vasodilation—the widening of blood vessels.

Found in: Broccoli, Brussel sprouts, asparagus, leafy greens such as collard, mustard, and turnip greens, bok choy, spinach, kale, Swiss chard, rainbow chard, and arugula.

BLUE/VIOLET

Superpower: Antioxidants, anthocyanins. May scavenge free radicals, improves neurological health, and supports vision and eye health.

Found in: Blueberries, blackberries, purple grapes, black grapes, plums, purple carrots, purple sweet potatoes, red onion, purple cabbage, eggplant, and purple cauliflower.

Now that we have stocked our refrigerator with healing foods, let's take a look at what to do next.

LET'S LOOK AT A SNAPSHOT OF A DAY OF VEGAN EATING

You now know how your food can be your "Farm-acy." You have seen the nutritive and healing power of foods. From what you have learned so far, think about how the following simple dishes are so nurturing and healing. Consider how your health is being supported by the the ingredients in each meal you make. How is each ingredient you eat contributing to help your body? Let's look at a sample menu for the day and what each ingredient is doing to increase our health.

```
A DAY OF EATING VEGAN SAMPLE MENU
```

BREAKFAST PARFAIT

Ingredients:

- Coconut non-dairy yogurt (Probiotics)
- Cinnamon (Blood pressure and blood glucose control)
- Raspberries (Anti-oxidants)
- Sprinkle of cereal (Vitamin D supplemented, fiber)

CARDAMOM COFFEE

I love the ritual of coffee in the morning. If you do not want the caffeine, you can certainly enjoy decaffeinated coffee. It is wonderful to grind the beans yourself, and inhale the smell of the freshly ground beans. You can find inexpensive coffee grinders online. It is so much more rewarding to make and savor your own coffee than to pay a store for a pesticide and GMO cup of Joe in a plastic hormone disrupting container. Your cost savings by making coffee at home will add up quickly to pay for your grinder and coffee supply investment. I prefer to use the pour-over method to prepare one cup at a time. You can also use a coffee press, which is easy and is single-cup or multi-cup serving depending on size, or you can percolate coffee in a coffee percolator, which is fun to watch and provides an even richer flavor.

You can add your spices into the coffee grounds and then proceed with making the coffee. If you like, you can add the spices directly to your cup for a single serving.

Ingredients:
- Freshly ground coffee (Riboflavin, vitamin B2)
- ¼ tsp ground Cardamom (Antioxidant)
- ¼ tsp ground Cinnamon (Blood pressure and blood glucose control) *

Please note: Do not stop taking your blood pressure and insulin medications because you are adding cinnamon into your foods. You will need to get your blood pressure and glucose history levels checked by your doctor, who may then make any appropriate medication changes if needed.

Preparation:
- Prepare your coffee with the spices mixed in the coffee grounds, or directly in your cup.
- Add oat milk instead of a dairy creamer.
- If you like your coffee sweetened, experiment with a little maple syrup or agave as a sweetener.
- Again, you can experiment further, adding fresh mint leaves, a drop of peppermint essential oil, or a dash of vanilla extract to your coffee, too.

MISO SOUP

Ingredients:

- Miso paste mixed with filtered water (Prebiotic)
- GMO-free organic firm tofu (Protein, amino acids)
- Dulse seaweed flakes (Thyroid support, fiber, minerals)
- Scallions (Anti-oxidant, anti-bacterial, fiber)

> **PRO TIP**: Don't be afraid to go "off the recipe" to make a dish your own. Get creative, and as you taste new spices, add them into your recipes. Making buckwheat pancakes? Why not add cacao? What could you add to personalize the healing dish you are preparing to make it even more hearty? For the miso soup recipe above, you could add turmeric with black pepper (anti-inflammatory, cancer fighting), radish slices and other veggies like frozen peas.

HOMEMADE HUMMUS

Try making your own customized hummus with cumin and lemon, rosemary and lemon, or a spice of your liking such as smoked paprika or chili powder. How might these ingredients in this dish be healthy nutrition for our body? As you prepare foods, consider the health benefits of the individual ingredients. How might a miso soup and hummus meal seed and feed our gut bacteria?

Ingredients:

- Dried chickpeas, soaked per directions (Protein and fiber)

- Tahini (Anti-inflammatory, anti-oxidant)

- Rosemary (Anti-viral)

- Lemon juice, freshly squeezed (Vitamin C, alkalinizing)

- Olive Oil (Anti-inflammatory, anti-oxidant)

- Garlic (Vitamins and anti-oxidants)

- Garnish with scallions (Vitamins K and C)

PRO TIP: Slice up red, green and yellow bell peppers, celery, or carrots to dip into your hummus or salsas instead of chips for an even healthier option.

"BOWL OF GOODNESS,"
ALSO KNOWN AS A "BUDDHA BOWL"

A "Bowl of Goodness" is a great way to use up miscellaneous veggies in your fridge. Key ingredients are the base of rice, or quinoa and tofu, and you can add on from there. You can really make this Buddha Bowl into your own custom creation!

- Start with a healthy brown rice or quinoa base (Protein)

- Cubes of baked sweet potato (Fiber and prebiotics)

- Sauerkraut (Probiotic)

- Sliced, pre-cooked beets (Fiber)

- Beans (Prebiotic, fiber, protein)

- Caramelized leeks (Vitamin A, C, K and fiber)

- Caramelized onion (Antioxidant)

- Fresh chopped garlic (Antioxidant)

- Assorted chopped fresh veggies such as carrots or peppers,

- Tofu (Protein) marinated for a few hours in grated ginger, (Anti-inflammatory) and scallions, (Fiber) tossed with low sodium organic tamari sauce

Garnishes:
- Nutritional Yeast (B12)

- Fresh mint (Anti-inflammatory, as well as breath freshening after those garlic and onions!)

- Cilantro leaves (Cleansing, de-toxifying)

PRO TIP: Some people have a gene that makes cilantro taste like soap to them, so offer the cilantro as a side dish to add as desired instead of mixing it into your recipe.

PRO TIP: Add an ounce (a small palmful) of raw, unsalted, nutritious, protein-packed, anti-inflammatory Omega 3 walnuts into your "Bowl of Goodness," on your oatmeal or cereal, salads, or to have on the go as a nutritious snack each day.

HOW TO MAKE IT EASIER TO EAT
VEGAN/WHOLE FOOD PLANT-BASED (WFPB)

Resource the 21-Day Vegan Kickstart meal planning program brought to you by the Physicians Committee for Responsible Medicine (PCRM) at www.21DayKickstart.org

- Having fresh, ready-to-eat produce in the refrigerator is help-ful for a snack that is easy to grab and go. Keep a few favorite and nutritious go-to snacks on hand, prepped, and ready to eat in baggies in the refrigerator for convenience when hunger or cravings arise. Having easily accessible and prepped snacks can help as a go-to when you may have otherwise made a not so healthy choice for that snack. Step away from the chips, no matter what those pesky taste buds are screaming!

- Add in fruits throughout your day as snacks. You can place a self-contained snack like an apple, banana, orange or clemen-tines in a baggie with a paper towel in your tote bag or purse for a healthy snack anytime.

- When you cook, prepare large portions of pasta sauce, soup, or stew, which you can freeze, reheat and add to fresh-made pasta or rice, along with fresh herbs like basil for garnish. Batch cooking saves time and is great in the event you have surprise guests or need to make a meal on the go—you will always have a nice, easy to make, stress-free home cooked meal at the ready.

- Washing and prepping produce at home is almost always less expensive than purchasing pre-cut and pre-washed produce. Prepped fruits and veggies can be stored in jars, storage bags, or food storage containers.

- If you do not have the space at your home for a garden, could you join a local community garden or even grow some herbs in a pot on your windowsill? Could you visit the local farms from your farmer's market to see where your food comes from? Is it possible to go and pick the fruit or vegetable yourself on your visit? This would be a really nice "field trip" for the family to enjoy.

- Buddy up! Get a buddy to join in with you as your support. Go out on a "field trip" to a new area. Make it a treat to go to a new vegan restaurant that is getting rave reviews. This is a great way to see what types of foods and ingredient combinations are on the menu, so you can try adding your own signature to them when you recreate them with your own personal touch at home.

- You could make a "vegan challenge" with your buddy, the goal being to turn new habits into a lifestyle, not only for you, but your buddy as well. Can you have a contest with your buddy on recreating this dish? You could incorporate some friends as "judges," and this would also serve to introduce them to vegan cooking. The more folks you have in your circle who are working on their health, the better you will be supported, too.

- The next time you go to the grocery store, take a look in other people's carts. What are they buying to put into and on their bodies? Is their cart full of packaged and processed foods, meats, snack foods, soda and chemical-laden products, or is it full of nutritious fruits, vegetables, rice, beans, seeds, and nuts? What kind of burden does their body have to carry to clear the toxic load in the products they are purchasing, using, and eating?

- While at the grocery store, look at the ingredients in a bag of your (ex) favorite fried potato or corn chips. How fast do the calories add up? 10 chips equal 200 calories? Come ON! No judgments here, but who only has 10 chips? How many calories do you find in an entire bag, which is the normal for someone to eat mindlessly before they know they did it? (Again, no judgments! I have been there!) Let's say it is 600 calories, which would only be 3 servings in the bag. It would take a *lot* of time exercising on the treadmill to work this off. Is it worth it? Not only would a person gain weight eating this way, it is a setup for obesity, diabetes, cancer, cardiac disease, and other diseases. What is the risk versus the fleeting reward for those silly taste buds? Health and longevity are dependent on quality nutrition from good food. Eating garbage can make you feel like garbage, too. Now let's put that bag down and select a healthier snack option!

WEEKLY HOMEWORK
[CHECK OFF WHEN COMPLETED]

☐ Watch the movie *Food, Inc.* (2009) online.

☐ Pick out one article from the "Suggested Reading" list below below and read it. Record your thoughts about the article in your journal.

☐ Suggested Reading for further information:

Chapter 44 of *Prevention of Chronic Disease by Means of Diet and Lifestyle Changes*
https://www.ncbi.nlm.nih.gov/books/NBK11795/

"Nutritional Update for Physicians: Plant-Based Diets"
http://www.thepermanentejournal.org/issues/2013/spring/5117-nutrition.html

Heart Disease and Stroke Statistics
https://doi.org/10.1161/CIR.0000000000000659

"Plant-Based Diet Reverses Vascular Endothelial Dysfunction in Patients with Peripheral Arterial Disease"
https://ijdrp.org/index.php/ijdrp/article/view/53

"Vegetarian diets and incidence of diabetes in the Adventist Health Study-2"
https://www.ncbi.nlm.nih.gov/pmc/articles/PMC3638849/#!po=14.4444

"Lifestyle changes CAN reverse coronary artery disease"

https://www.thelancet.com/journals/lancet/article/PII0140-6736(90)91656-U/fulltext

"The effects of plant-based diets on the body and the brain: a systematic review"

https://www.nature.com/articles/s41398-019-0552-0

Dietary fiber intake and risk of cardiovascular disease: systematic review and meta-analysis

https://www.bmj.com/content/347/bmj.f6879

Day 43: YOUR HEART TO SOUL DAILY JOURNAL

DATE: _____

DAILY WEIGHT: _____   A.M. GLUCOSE: _____

TODAY'S OVERALL FEELING OF WELLNESS:

1   2   3   4   5   6   7   8   9   10

INTENTION WORD FOR THE DAY: _____

TODAY I ACCOMPLISHED:

☐ Mindful breath work

☐ Mindful meditation (Duration _____)

☐ Joy & Meaning self-care activity: _____

3 THINGS I AM GRATEFUL FOR TODAY:

1.

2.

3.

WHAT'S ON YOUR MIND?

Day 44: YOUR HEART TO SOUL DAILY JOURNAL

DATE: _____

DAILY WEIGHT:_____ A.M. GLUCOSE:_____

TODAY'S OVERALL FEELING OF WELLNESS:

1   2   3   4   5   6   7   8   9   10

INTENTION WORD FOR THE DAY:_____

TODAY I ACCOMPLISHED:

☐ Mindful breath work

☐ Mindful meditation (Duration _____)

☐ Joy & Meaning self-care activity:_____

3 THINGS I AM GRATEFUL FOR TODAY:

1.

2.

3.

WHAT'S ON YOUR MIND?

Day 45: YOUR HEART TO SOUL DAILY JOURNAL

DATE: _____

DAILY WEIGHT:_____   A.M. GLUCOSE:_____

TODAY'S OVERALL FEELING OF WELLNESS:

1   2   3   4   5   6   7   8   9   10

INTENTION WORD FOR THE DAY:_____

TODAY I ACCOMPLISHED:

☐ Mindful breath work

☐ Mindful meditation (Duration _____)

☐ Joy & Meaning self-care activity:_____

3 THINGS I AM GRATEFUL FOR TODAY:

1.

2.

3.

WHAT'S ON YOUR MIND?

Day 46: YOUR HEART TO SOUL DAILY JOURNAL

DATE: _____

DAILY WEIGHT: _____ A.M. GLUCOSE: _____

TODAY'S OVERALL FEELING OF WELLNESS:

1   2   3   4   5   6   7   8   9   10

INTENTION WORD FOR THE DAY: _____

TODAY I ACCOMPLISHED:

☐ Mindful breath work

☐ Mindful meditation (Duration _____)

☐ Joy & Meaning self-care activity: _____

3 THINGS I AM GRATEFUL FOR TODAY:

1.

2.

3.

WHAT'S ON YOUR MIND?

Day 47: YOUR HEART TO SOUL DAILY JOURNAL

DATE: _____

DAILY WEIGHT:_____   A.M. GLUCOSE:_____

TODAY'S OVERALL FEELING OF WELLNESS:

1   2   3   4   5   6   7   8   9   10

INTENTION WORD FOR THE DAY:_____

TODAY I ACCOMPLISHED:

☐ Mindful breath work

☐ Mindful meditation (Duration _____)

☐ Joy & Meaning self-care activity:_____

3 THINGS I AM GRATEFUL FOR TODAY:

1.

2.

3.

WHAT'S ON YOUR MIND?

Day 48: YOUR HEART TO SOUL DAILY JOURNAL

DATE: _____

DAILY WEIGHT:_____ A.M. GLUCOSE:_____

TODAY'S OVERALL FEELING OF WELLNESS:

1   2   3   4   5   6   7   8   9   10

INTENTION WORD FOR THE DAY:_____

TODAY I ACCOMPLISHED:

☐ Mindful breath work

☐ Mindful meditation (Duration _____)

☐ Joy & Meaning self-care activity:_____

3 THINGS I AM GRATEFUL FOR TODAY:

1.

2.

3.

WHAT'S ON YOUR MIND?

Day 49: **YOUR HEART TO SOUL DAILY JOURNAL**

DATE: _____

DAILY WEIGHT: _____ A.M. GLUCOSE: _____

TODAY'S OVERALL FEELING OF WELLNESS:

1   2   3   4   5   6   7   8   9   10

INTENTION WORD FOR THE DAY: _____

TODAY I ACCOMPLISHED:

☐ Mindful breath work

☐ Mindful meditation (Duration _____)

☐ Joy & Meaning self-care activity: _____

3 THINGS I AM GRATEFUL FOR TODAY:

1.

2.

3.

WHAT'S ON YOUR MIND?

Week 8:

EVERYDAY THINGS YOU CAN DO TO ENHANCE YOUR HEALTH

Our bodies know when we are helping them. They feel better as we strive to reach and then maintain homeostasis. We have all the benefits of scientifically proven Western medicine, yet Western medicine alone leaves out the additional things we can do daily to support our health and immunity. Western medicine offers only a part of the entire wellness spectrum. We can also bolster our health holistically. This means that in addition to the necessary treatments and medicines prescribed by physicians, we can complete our wellness plan by looking to other, less known but effective ways of healing to help us get well, feel better, and live longer.

Below you will find information to add into your health and wellness toolkit. As we move through topics in this book, it's important to be open to consider different approaches to healing and feeling your best. My goal here is to make you aware that these other wellness options exist, so you can add them in to your health and wellness plan. These healing modalities can be layered together as a part of your self-care. You can do everything if you want to. Consider this chapter your "Health Smorgasbord!"

AYURVEDA

We can use holistic Ayurvedic healing practices to complement our Western medicine treatment plan to help us optimize our health. Ayurveda is the healing sister science to Yoga. Ayurveda means "The Science of Life" in Sanskrit language. The healing practices of Ayurveda originated in India thousands of years ago. Ayurveda encompasses traditional Indian wellness practices and techniques as a guide to live everyday life while honoring our own individual constitution or "Dosha." Ayurveda presents general wellness practices and then if you would like to study further, there are practices tailored to your unique Dosha; your blend of elements. For fun you can take a Dosha test here to see what your Dosha is: https://www.banyanbotanicals.com/info/dosha-quiz

WHAT CAN WE LEARN FROM AYURVEDA?

Have you heard the saying: "You are what you eat!"? Well, if you think about it, aren't you actually more of what you *digest*? The food you put in your mouth is taken into your body for nourishment and what your body does not need is then evacuated, so you really are what you eat *and* digest. In Ayurveda it is important to support our digestive system, the base of our immunity. Our gut is filled with good bacteria called the "microbiome" which has many beneficial functions and plays a key role in immune system development and protection against disease. These gut bacteria regulate immune cell homeostasis. Signals from intestinal bacteria alert and inform our immune cells and help regulate pro and anti-inflammatory immune system responses. It is important for our immunity to keep these gut bacteria healthy. Ayurveda goes beyond "seed and feed" to further support our gut bacteria.

A big reason to optimize our microbiome holistically is because we have created antibiotic resistant bacterial "Superbugs" through our overuse of antibiotics in our animals that we eat, and in what is prescribed to us. When we take antibiotics, in addition to killing the bad bacteria, good bacteria are killed, too. These bad Superbugs then take over and can make us very ill. This unbalanced state in our gut bacteria is called dysbiosis.

PRO TIP: If you do have to take antibiotics, support your gut health by "seeding" (with probiotics) and "feeding" (with prebiotics). Do take your prescription for the full amount of antibiotic prescribed by your doctor. Stopping before completion of your prescription may allow the bad bugs to grow back even stronger and you may get sick again.

HOW TO HELP OUR DIGESTION, THE AYURVEDIC WAY

First thing in the morning after using the bathroom and weighing yourself:

TONGUE SCRAPING

What the heck is tongue scraping? Use a copper or stainless steel tongue scraper (found online) which cleans toxins off of the tongue that have risen from the GI tract overnight. Tongue scraping stimulates the peristalsis (movements) of the gastrointestinal tract, promoting a bowel movement. Note: If you have a sensitive gag reflex, instead of tongue scraping, try oil pulling, below.

OIL PULLING

After or in lieu of tongue scraping, use 1 teaspoon of organic coconut oil, which is anti-fungal and bacteriostatic. Swirl and swish the oil in your mouth for a few minutes. This cleans the oral cavity. Spit the oil into a tissue and then discard the tissue into the trash. Don't spit it into the sink or toilet because it will clog the pipes. And most importantly: don't swallow the coconut oil, because it contains all of those toxins in it that you just pulled from your oral cavity.

GARGLE

Gargle with warm salt water morning and evening if you don't have organic coconut oil. Gargling moistens your mucous membranes, which is important, especially if you are a snorer or breathe through your mouth and it gets dry. Gargling stimulates the vagus nerve because the muscles of the vocal cords are connected to the vagus nerve. This is a great way to improve vagal tone and increase heart rate variability, which is a sign of a healthy nervous system.

MORNING HYDRATION

After oil pulling or gargling, drink a glass of filtered room temperature lemon water taken all at once. Lemon water serves to stimulate the gastrointestinal tract, further helping along a morning bowel movement. Lemon water creates alkalinity, thought to be an unfriendly environment for disease in your body, even though the lemon is acidic in your mouth.

> PRO TIP: Lemon water or other citrus water is not to be sipped all day, because the acid in the citrus may damage the enamel on your teeth, weakening them and promoting cavities. Always rinse your mouth after eating or drinking a citrus fruit/juice.

ROOM TEMPERATURE BEVERAGES

Room temperature or warm drinks work together with the digestive system. According to Ayurvedic teachings, drinking iced or cold drinks puts out the digestive fire. It throws a cold, wet blanket onto the fire of our stomach acids, making the stomach acids less strong when the stomach is trying to digest our foods. Think of it this way: If we were to build a roaring fire, then threw a soggy wet blanket on top of it, would that fire be able to burn as hot or as bright? We want to help our digestion along as much as possible to promote smooth elimination, and to create less strain on our body and heart when processing food into fuel.

DRY BRUSH

Dry brush your skin with a loofah or brushing mitt prior to your shower to increase lymphatic flow, remove dried skin cells, and stimulate collagen renewal. Collagen is the most abundant protein in your body. It is one of the major building blocks of skin, vessels, tissues and bones. Collagen is the "glue" that holds all these things together. The word collagen comes from the Greek word "kólla," which means glue.

Dry brush in circular motions from your hands and feet towards your heart. Notice how you may feel invigorated and your skin may tingle after dry brushing. Your skin may feel smoother as a result of removing dry, flaky skin. After dry brushing, and then a warm shower, your skin is free of dead skin cells, your pores are open and now ready to receive a slathering of organic coconut oil as a natural moisturizer without any toxic additives.

UPLIFT YOUR BODY AND MIND WITH THE FOLLOWING, WHICH COMPLEMENT AYURVEDA AND WESTERN MEDICINE

ESSENTIAL OILS

Apply or diffuse organic essential oils for uplifting mood aromatherapy. You can use essential oils instead of toxic chemical and artificial fragrance-filled perfumes or colognes. Essential oil companies have created blends you can try, or like spices, you can create your own blends based on what benefits you would like to receive and how you would like to feel and smell that day. You can also layer the oils on your body, to make a custom scent for the day. It is fun to experiment!

I encourage you to do your own online research on which essential oils are recommended for which ailments and what way is best to use them. Try a very small amount at first to ensure you have no allergic reaction. I have highlighted some oils I like in the "Boutique" section in my website www.hearttosoulcw.com.

> PRO TIP: Make sure you dilute the essential oil with a diluting "carrier oil" such as almond oil if instructed, when topically using to avoid a burn from direct skin application of an undiluted essential oil. Some oils are photosensitive, such as citrus oils, and may cause skin burning or skin discoloration.

MEDITATE

Do your breathing exercises and meditation as a consistent part of your morning routine to help put your mind at ease, calm your body, and clear space in your mind for the day ahead. You can apply your essential oils to set a relaxing mood for your meditation.

GROUND YOURSELF IN POSITIVITY

Think positive thoughts. Catch yourself if you are having negative thoughts and move to thoughts of gratitude. Having an attitude of positivity can increase our telomeres, the end of our genes, promoting a longer life. Recall the case of the Twins, and how their lifestyle and environment activated their individual positive or negative gene expression. The energy we put out to the world, such as happiness, draws that kind of energy back to us. This is called the "Law of

Attraction." Make a pact with yourself to stop those negative thoughts and turn them into positives. Your positivity will flow outwards to positively affect others. When you combine positive thoughts with your breathing techniques, you assume control of your stress response. Enabling this relaxation response will move your body to a calmer state, which can positively impact your blood pressure (lowering it) and heart rate (slowing it down) which are beneficial for the heart. Lower blood pressure means the heart doesn't have to pump as hard against constricted arteries to get your blood through your circulation. Fewer heart beats means that the heart can get the job done without efforting so much. We all want that!

MOVE YOUR BODY

First, see your doctor for approval before starting an exercise program of any kind. Ask your doctor if Yoga or Tai Chi or simply walking to move your body every day is helpful for your current health condition.

Sitting is the new smoking in relation to wellness. If you reference a vibrant older person you know, chances are they are not sitting; they are up, moving around, and busy living their lives. Like the long living communities in the "Blue Zones," my neighbor is 93, and this little lady is always busy! She gets up every morning and sweeps her porch of leaves, still drives her car to do her grocery shopping, has a little above ground pool she paddles around in, is active with her senior center helping others, and has a loving family, who comes to visit her often at her own home. She eats healthfully and has an upbeat attitude. She is her own mini Blue Zone! We can learn a lot from her example.

I remember once in one of my earliest yoga classes, my teacher Jean said: "Let's all sit down on our mats on the floor and then get up. If you cannot sit down and then get up from the floor when you are 30 or 40, what are you going to do when you are 80?" That was an "Ah-Ha!" moment for us!

For a wonderful before and after story, of regained health, see www.fatmanrants.com for Tim Kaufman's health journey.

"EAT PLANTS AND MOVE YOUR BODY. ALL YA GOTTA DO IS A LITTLE MORE THAN YA DID YESTERDAY!"

—TIM KAUFMAN, author and public speaker

GRATITUDE

Take time each day for prayer, intention, and offering thanks, and record in the space provided in your daily journal. Close your eyes. Visualize positive things manifesting for you, and give thanks for them now, as if they have already happened. Visualization is very powerful in helping us to achieve our goals. This book you are reading was my own visualization before I wrote it. I am grateful you found it, and I hope you are receiving valuable information from it. Please do share any takeaways you may have with me. I would love to hear from you! Please feel free to connect with me on my Instagram account: @hearttosoulcw. I am so grateful for you and how much light you are shining into the world!

HEALTHY EATING

Notice how and when you eat. Do you stand at a kitchen counter or sit in front of a TV, mindlessly eating mouthfuls of snacks, or are you sitting down enjoying healthy and thoughtfully prepared food, slowly chewing and savoring each bite? Are you eating when you are not hungry? Do you eat certain things for comfort? Notice patterns of behavior you may have around your food.

TEA

Drink green, black, and herbal teas for overall health and digestion. Teas, especially green teas, work for us as antioxidants, and help to decrease inflammation. Green tea is a great alternative if you do not like coffee, and it has less caffeine than coffee.

> **PRO TIP**: Add fresh mint to your tea or a squeeze of lemon to enhance flavor. Toss in a peeled chunk of fresh ginger for digestion.

HERBS AND SPICES

Remember to explore and add spices and herbs and even a seaweed like dulse flakes to your dishes. Sprinkle your foods with garlic and onion powders, smoked paprika, curry, cumin, turmeric combined with black pepper, ginger, rosemary, sage, thyme, oregano and so many others. Explore and try new taste combinations, all of which kick up the health level of your food, without adding calories. I encourage you to search online for the spices above, find out their healing benefits and start to experiment with them in your meal creations.

OTHER WAYS TO ENHANCE THE BODY/MIND/SPIRIT CONNECTION

By incorporating additional holistic healing techniques, we are complementing our Western medical plan to offer our heart and body additional healing modalities to address areas such as body energy, stress release, foods as medicine, and socialization, which have the power to optimize, heal, and positively impact our overall health and well-being.

WHAT CAN CRYSTALS DO?

Before we talk about the healing energy and power of crystals, I want to ask you a question: When you blow a dog whistle, do you as a human hear the frequency of the whistle sound? Humans cannot hear the sound, yet dogs can. This shows us that just because something is not tangible before our eyes and ears doesn't mean it is not present.

Science has incorporated the energetic use of crystals into technology, due to their ability to amplify and transmit energy. Liquid crystal displays (LCDs) project images, such as those found in flat TV screen monitors, computers, digital watches, quartz watches, and telephones.

A famous IBM scientist, Marcel Vogel, worked with the healing energy potential of crystals. He perceived that crystals worked with an energy in the unlimited infinite domain, can serve as a radio transmitter, a memory element, a transceiver, (transmitting and receiving communication) and as a computer that delivers small doses of natural radiation to the body, using a natural element. He created crystal wands using a special "Vogel Cut" for his experimental techniques with crystals as energy healers.

Christiane Northrup, M.D., author of *Women's Bodies, Women's Wisdom* writes that the fascia (connective tissue) of your body "functions as a liquid crystalline matrix highly affected by your level of hydration." "…And it's the crystalline properties of connective tissue (as well as of bones and teeth) that enable it to transmit information and energy instantaneously throughout the body." In other words: make sure you are getting plenty of water, at least 8 glasses a day, (unless you have a medical fluid restriction) which will enhance the ability of your body to communicate with itself and to function at an optimal level.

Reflection Questions: www.usgs.gov states the human body on average is composed of 55-60% water. Take a moment to consider how the ocean tides are affected by the cycles of the moon and gravity. Aren't our bodies little "individual oceans" of water? Might our body energy be affected by how hydrated we are? Have you ever experienced people not quite "acting like themselves" during a full moon? Could it be that their energy was off from the gravitational pull of the moon on the fluids in their body? These are reflection questions to introduce you to the potential power of crystal energy use and to open your mind to new ways of perceiving energy.

Crystals, energetic sources from the earth, serve as talismans we can use to help us heal. We can assign them "work," empowering them by "charging" them and caring for them. After "cleansing" a crystal monthly in the light of the full moon, you can charge it by assigning it "work" that you would like help with.

I want to encourage you to explore the healing power of crystals on your own. This healing work is something deeply personal and based on your unique needs. I have provided book recommendations for reference in the "Resource Boutique" at the end of your book to help you on your crystal journey.

You may also search online "Crystals for..." inserting whatever you are looking for in a crystal, such as "Crystals for arthritis" or "Crystals for the heart." See what comes up for you. There is a surprising amount of information on the healing power of crystals.

> PRO TIP: You can make a little space for your crystals and incorporate other talismans such as feathers, shells, driftwood, pretty rocks, little statues, and anything that makes you feel at peace. This could be a space by your meditation area, or a place that you come to frequently during your day for inspiration, or journaling. Even a windowsill will do. Cultivate this space as a special place for you to find joy and calm. Note: Crystals should not be placed in direct sunlight.

SOUND HEALING THERAPY

Sound healings are wonderful to meditate to or to have on in the background while you work. Some sound healing therapies to look for are the sounds of singing bowls, gong baths, sound baths, low Hertz frequency sound, sounds of nature like waves crashing, or rain falling on leaves, and Solfeggio music, which contains an energetic vibrational sound wavelength. You will have your own preferences of the sounds and tones you like to hear, so doing that research to see what feels healing to you is important. You can find many free sound healing therapies to listen to on the internet. Sample different types of sound healing therapies until you find which types of sounds you prefer. One of the crystal bowl sound healing frequencies for the heart is 528 Hz (Hertz).

ENERGY HEALING WITH REIKI AND ACUPUNCTURE

Explore other alternative methods like the energy healing of Reiki (a hands-off energetic exchange for healing) and Acupuncture, which is another complemental therapy to Western medicine using needles in energetic points in the body, which correlate to the area needing treatment. There are other forms of energy healing as well. I encourage you to research these modalities online to explore what works best for you. You can even learn to use Reiki healing practices on yourself. One of my nurse colleagues performed Reiki on me, which felt so energetically healing. I could feel my body vibrating differently after her hands-off Reiki healing treatment. Again, this is something unique for you and your health needs, so why not take a look at these offerings and see what works best as a health and healing complement for you.

SUSTAINABLE CLOTHING

Why are we talking about clothing, you may ask? Notice what you are wearing today. Is it made from natural fibers? What material is next to your skin? Are you wearing cotton, or are you wearing things made from a man-made synthetic fiber? How might wearing a synthetic fabric disable the ability of our skin to breathe, adding strain on the body as yet another layer it is fighting against to maintain homeostasis? Your clothing lives next to the largest organ of your body—your skin. As much as possible, consider buying organic cotton, especially for your undergarments. It all goes back to decreasing the toxic load on your body and enhancing your overall wellness, which in turn makes the heart and all of your organs function closer to that state of homeostasis we are aiming for. This is true for all products we use on a daily basis.

We are working on feeling great, and that includes our physical presentation to the world. Do you buy new clothes all the time? Do you pick out designer labels? Would you like to look great, feel good about the environment and save money? Clothing manufacturing creates a strain on our environment in its unhealthy production. How does this lead back to your heart? Pollution in the air we breathe ultimately goes into our lungs, and that means there is less room for clean oxygen, that your heart loves and needs.

Sustainable fashion, or eco-fashion, is a movement aimed at changing how people buy clothing and how the fashion industry can function in a more ecologically friendly manner. Sustainable fashion is closely aligned with taking a hard look at our environment and at social justice goals. If we recycle bottles and paper products into usable commodities, why not do the same with clothing? What happens to synthetic, man-made fabric used in making clothing after the person no longer wears the garment? Is it easily biodegradable or does it end up in a landfill? Why not repurpose what we wear?

> PRO TIP: Save money by shopping at vintage stores, thrift shops, consignment shops, or online second-hand clothing sites where

you can find stunning, unique, one-of-a-kind garments. Sometimes people wear something once, then sell or donate it to these kinds of stores. Garage sales and flea markets are also a great way to help reduce manufacturing, save money, and find a piece that no one else will be wearing this year. You'll look fantastic and Mother Earth will appreciate your reduced environmental footprint.

In kind, can you give away clothes to help someone out? Can you donate things to stores that resell, or to a flea market if you are not using them? Could you have a "swap meet" with friends, everyone bringing things they no longer want, to trade or give away?

Challenge: Take inventory of your clothing items. Are they bringing you joy or is it time to pass them on to make room for new items? Some of you may want to keep items for sentimental reasons, even though they are out of style or do not fit. That's great. The goal is to relieve your life of those clothes that are burdening you and causing clutter in your environment. Maybe you even don't "feel" right in those old clothes. If they do not bring you joy and you have other clothes to wear, pass them on or donate them, a la Marie Kondo's book, *The Life-Changing Magic of Tidying Up*. As a bonus, someone else may really need, appreciate, and enjoy what you gave away.

BODY AND BEAUTY

Let's take a walk to your bathroom. Pull out the products you use every day: toothpaste, soap, shampoo, hair conditioner, antiperspirant, deodorant, mouthwash, body lotion, creams, makeup, lipstick or lip balm, perfume, nail polish, nail polish remover, and cologne. Now take a look at each of their ingredient lists.

Do you know what the ingredients in your body care products are? Can you pronounce them? Are they organic? Are they found in nature? Would you spoon the ingredients into your mouth? If you wouldn't put it in your mouth, it shouldn't be put on your skin or anywhere where it will be absorbed in your body.

Your skin is the largest external organ of your body. Your skin's pores allow it to absorb what you put on it, directly into your body. What you put on your skin is as important as what you put in your mouth. Some ingredients found in antiperspirants, lotions, shampoos, bath and body products, makeup, and cleaning products may contain harmful chemicals that can cause Alzheimer's disease, cancers, and serve as hormone disruptors. These chemicals can interfere with our hormone regulation, and can also cause diseases, birth defects, and developmental disorders. Examples of hormone disruptors are chemicals found in some plastics and pesticides. I encourage you to do your own research on the chemicals in your bath and body products. Would you eat Aluminum Zirconium Trichlorohydrex Gly, Cyclopentasiloxane, Dimethicone, Talc, and PPG-14 Butyl Ether? I found these and many more toxic ingredients in an antiperspirant I no longer use. That was only one of the many products I was using daily that were full of toxic chemicals. Imagine the toxic load our bodies try to fend off each day to maintain homeostasis, while what we are simultaneously putting *on* and *into* our body is hurting our body.

Our bodies *want* to detox; sweating is a way for the body to cool itself and to release toxins. Consider making the switch from antiperspirants to *deodorants*. Deodorants help eliminate some of the odor-causing bacteria, while still allowing your body to perspire naturally. I switched to companies with healthy products I believe in. As a *Heart to Soul Cardiac Wellness* reader, some of these companies whose products I love will gift you with a discount. Please refer to my website www.hearttosoulcw.com in the "Boutique" header for a listing of companies offering discount to *Heart to Soul Cardiac Wellness* readers.

WEEKLY HOMEWORK
(CHECK OFF WHEN COMPLETED)

☐ It is time to get our detective hats on again. Look at ingredients in your self-care and cleaning products. Switch out one item at a time with a healthier alternative, starting this week. Replace items as you run out with new healthier alternatives. Toothpaste, soap, laundry detergent, home cleaning supplies, lotion, creams, fragrances, makeup, take a look at all of it. How might this cumulatively be adding a burden to your body? A good rule of thumb is: *"If you cannot pronounce it, you probably shouldn't be wearing it or using it!"* Be a sleuth on those crazy ingredients you cannot pronounce, and look them up. Are the ingredients healing or are they a chemical that will add additional toxic burden to your body?

☐ Research and find a couple of stores that carry crystals. Look at the crystals, feel their presence, touch them, note what they are used for and see if one pops out at you. What crystal spoke to you and why? What energy are they empowering you with? Did you feel moved to purchase it? Why? Document in your journal. If you cannot find a store nearby, you can find lots of sites on Instagram and online. Research which crystal would be best for your healing needs and how to use it.

- [ ] Prepare a list of wellness topics that you would like to address with essential oil healing. Research which essential oil would be best for healing and how to use it. You can topically wear oils, or diffuse them with a special diffuser which gently mists the air with the oils. Make sure you are using the oil the correct way.

- [ ] Research non-toxic home cleaning products. Research how you can "Do It Yourself" using items for cleaning such as lemon juice or apple cider vinegar or essential oils instead of using chemically laden commercial cleaning products.

Day 50: YOUR HEART TO SOUL DAILY JOURNAL

DATE: _____

DAILY WEIGHT:_____ A.M. GLUCOSE:_____

TODAY'S OVERALL FEELING OF WELLNESS:

1   2   3   4   5   6   7   8   9   10

INTENTION WORD FOR THE DAY:_____

TODAY I ACCOMPLISHED:

☐ Mindful breath work

☐ Mindful meditation (Duration _____)

☐ Joy & Meaning self-care activity:_____

3 THINGS I AM GRATEFUL FOR TODAY:

1.

2.

3.

WHAT'S ON YOUR MIND?

Day 51: **YOUR HEART TO SOUL DAILY JOURNAL**

DATE: _____

DAILY WEIGHT: _____   A.M. GLUCOSE: _____

TODAY'S OVERALL FEELING OF WELLNESS:

1   2   3   4   5   6   7   8   9   10

INTENTION WORD FOR THE DAY: _____

TODAY I ACCOMPLISHED:
- ☐ Mindful breath work
- ☐ Mindful meditation (Duration _____)
- ☐ Joy & Meaning self-care activity: _____

3 THINGS I AM GRATEFUL FOR TODAY:

1.

2.

3.

WHAT'S ON YOUR MIND?

Day 52: YOUR HEART TO SOUL DAILY JOURNAL

DATE: _____

DAILY WEIGHT: _____ **A.M. GLUCOSE:** _____

TODAY'S OVERALL FEELING OF WELLNESS:

1   2   3   4   5   6   7   8   9   10

INTENTION WORD FOR THE DAY: _____

TODAY I ACCOMPLISHED:

☐ Mindful breath work

☐ Mindful meditation (Duration _____)

☐ Joy & Meaning self-care activity: _____

3 THINGS I AM GRATEFUL FOR TODAY:

1.

2.

3.

WHAT'S ON YOUR MIND?

Day 53: **YOUR HEART TO SOUL DAILY JOURNAL**

DATE: _____

DAILY WEIGHT: _____ **A.M. GLUCOSE:** _____

TODAY'S OVERALL FEELING OF WELLNESS:

1   2   3   4   5   6   7   8   9   10

INTENTION WORD FOR THE DAY: _____

TODAY I ACCOMPLISHED:

☐ Mindful breath work

☐ Mindful meditation (Duration _____)

☐ Joy & Meaning self-care activity: _____

3 THINGS I AM GRATEFUL FOR TODAY:

1.

2.

3.

WHAT'S ON YOUR MIND?

Day 54: YOUR HEART TO SOUL DAILY JOURNAL

DATE: _____

DAILY WEIGHT: _____ A.M. GLUCOSE: _____

TODAY'S OVERALL FEELING OF WELLNESS:

1   2   3   4   5   6   7   8   9   10

INTENTION WORD FOR THE DAY: _____

TODAY I ACCOMPLISHED:

☐ Mindful breath work

☐ Mindful meditation (Duration _____)

☐ Joy & Meaning self-care activity: _____

3 THINGS I AM GRATEFUL FOR TODAY:

1.

2.

3.

WHAT'S ON YOUR MIND?

Day 55: **YOUR HEART TO SOUL DAILY JOURNAL**

DATE: _____

DAILY WEIGHT: _____ **A.M. GLUCOSE:** _____

TODAY'S OVERALL FEELING OF WELLNESS:

1   2   3   4   5   6   7   8   9   10

INTENTION WORD FOR THE DAY: _____

TODAY I ACCOMPLISHED:

☐ Mindful breath work

☐ Mindful meditation (Duration _____)

☐ Joy & Meaning self-care activity: _____

3 THINGS I AM GRATEFUL FOR TODAY:

1.

2.

3.

WHAT'S ON YOUR MIND?

Day 56: YOUR HEART TO SOUL DAILY JOURNAL

DATE: _____

DAILY WEIGHT: _____   **A.M. GLUCOSE:** _____

TODAY'S OVERALL FEELING OF WELLNESS:

1   2   3   4   5   6   7   8   9   10

INTENTION WORD FOR THE DAY: _____

TODAY I ACCOMPLISHED:

☐ Mindful breath work

☐ Mindful meditation (Duration _____)

☐ Joy & Meaning self-care activity: _____

3 THINGS I AM GRATEFUL FOR TODAY:

1.

2.

3.

WHAT'S ON YOUR MIND?

Week 9:

YOU ARE WHAT YOU THINK... AND WHAT YOU DON'T!

Check-in: Remember when we asked at the start of our time together, "What are your health goals?" How are you progressing toward those goals? Are you finding that you have established a wellness routine each day? Is it beginning to feel like a daily habit now? Are you consistently showing up for yourself? How are you feeling overall? Are you allowing yourself compassion? How does your heart energy feel? What does your graph look like from your daily charting?

Let's take a little test called "The Lemon Test." All you need for this test is your imagination. Ready? Here we go!

Imagine you are in your kitchen holding a big yellow lemon. You can tell by feeling it that this plump lemon is very juicy inside. Imagine putting that lemon on a plate, taking out your sharp knife, and slicing the lemon in half. There is a lot of juice on the plate after you cut into the lemon. Pick up one of the halves of the lemon. Now imagine that you tilt your head back as you squeeze the juice from the lemon directly into your mouth.

Did you just salivate? Did you generate a large amount of saliva in your mouth? There was no lemon, yet you produced saliva.

> This example was to show you how much our thoughts can influence our body.

Let's look at how we may be affected by thoughts and emotions, because they have important implications for our overall physical and mental well-being.

Swedish psychiatrist Elisabeth Kubler-Ross, author of the classic book *On Death and Dying*, cites five stages of grief: denial, anger, bargaining, depression and acceptance. As a cardiac patient, you may have added on "shock" as you heard your initial diagnosis, and "frustration" that this happened to you. You may feel slighted when you are waved off by others who tell you that "You'll be fine." You may have anger about the inconvenience of illness in your life, and fear of the unknown and what may happen to you in the future. These grief stages and emotions are fluid; you can move back and forth between them. You might feel like a slinky going back and forth, and at the same time feel like a wheel spinning.

Honoring the grief process and shedding tears can cleanse you and create an opening for you to gather yourself to face what is on the other side of this challenge. After all, it's in darkness is when we can best see light. We can't see stars in the daytime. We can get blocked by circumstances of our trauma, and working through this is a process. Everything happens for our soul maturity and that requires living in the experience, and working through it, even if it gets messy and gives us more than we think we can handle. These messy moments we have from our emotions are our life teachers.

"STRENGTH GROWS IN THE MOMENTS WHEN YOU THINK YOU CAN'T GO ON BUT YOU KEEP GOING ANYWAY."

—ED MYLETT, entrepreneur, business coach

You are on the precipice of big change by activating the information in this book into your life. It can be scary, and I want to take a moment to address fear.

Fear causes us to contract, withdraw, and freeze. Fear can cause inaction and immobility. Fear, and his brother "Worry" waste a lot of our time and emotional energy on something that may *never happen*. Transitioning over fear allows for the freedom to move forward.

Fear to change is the number one thing that kills all dreams and stops all growth. Fear stops us from progressing, trying something new, or attempting the unknown or unfamiliar. This is because we like to stay in that comfort zone of what we are familiar with and what we know.

"I TOOK A "FEAR OF FLYING" CLASS, AND I ALWAYS MISSED THE CLASS, BECAUSE I WAS ALWAYS FLYING."

—SARA BLAKELY, founder/owner of SPANX

Like a butterfly struggling to break out of its cocoon, you can't improve and be different if you aren't willing to endure the difficulty of change from being a caterpillar to pushing your way out of the cocoon as a butterfly. The struggle to get out of the cocoon is what gives the butterfly strength in its wings to fly on to its new exciting life. Dare to make changes and see what new things open up for you or come into your life. By shifting to an optimistic perspective, you are changing the vibration of your energy, and that will now align with new things coming to you with the same elevated energy, using "The Law of Attraction."

Give yourself permission to grow, and to experience this abundance. If something doesn't work out, this is a redirection for another opportunity. Maybe that path wouldn't have worked out so well, had we truly gone down it.

Rejection is redirection.

Rejection also serves as protection.

The obstacle IS the path.

I was talking to a friend about the concept of the obstacle being the path and I asked her what she would do if she had a boulder plunked down in the middle of the road in front of her. She said she would climb over it. Well, that was not the answer I thought she would give. I would think a person would walk around the boulder, on either side of it, but this example shows us how people choose different paths given their obstacles, and what we discover on these paths teaches us.

There is tremendous fear of the unknown, especially if you have suffered a health challenge. What will happen to me? Can my illness happen again? What is going to happen to my family? These are valid questions.

It's vital that you gather up all support in whatever way best serves you—and from all directions, gather your emotional support beams: family, friends, coaches, your faith leaders, your medical team, your therapist, neighbors, music, your journal, your yoga teachers, your crystals, your hobbies, and books. I have curated a library of books to support you in the "Resource Boutique" at the back of this book.

You have people in your corner to help you overcome this fear. Take a step back, look at your fear and reflect on what it is teaching you. What do you need to know about it? What obstacle is the fear shining a spotlight on? Then, physically and mentally, practice not allowing fear to bubble up, because *you have a plan with this book.* Fear and worry take the energy that could otherwise be used positively for constructive purposes. Your fears are valid, and you can acknowledge them, and by taking steps toward your health and well-being, you are moving further away from the situations you are fearful of.

"IF YOU WAIT FOR THE FEAR TO GO AWAY, THE OPPORTUNITY WILL GO AWAY, TOO."

—LESLIE BLODGETT, entrepreneur

Think to yourself: "I accept myself unconditionally, right now." Your health challenge was an obstacle put here to teach you, and because you have had this experience, it puts you closer to self-introspection. Accept every surgical scar, every test result, every medical appointment, you had, all of it. These are largely behind you now. They are evidence of your fight, and they are in the rear view mirror in the vehicle that is your life. You are the driver and you are looking through the front windshield at the future. You are here, now, and wherever you are in this moment you can begin again with hope.

HOW CAN WE LIVE FEARLESSLY?

LET GO OF THE NEED TO PLEASE ANYONE
This can lead to resentment because you are not pleasing yourself.

LET GO OF THE NEED TO BE IN CONTROL
With the effort of inspired intentions and actions first (doing the work necessary to get a goal accomplished), allow for the Universe's higher good to partner up with you to make it happen. Put positive thoughts and visualizations out to the Universe so it can help you manifest your dreams. Remember you can engage the "Law of Attraction" any time.

- Ask (Law of Attraction and Prayer)
- Believe (Visualization)
- Receive (Manifestation)

- Gratitude (Honor your gift with thanks and appreciation)
- Achieve (Use this gift to help others)

TAKE INVENTORY OF YOUR CIRCLE OF FRIENDS AND FAMILY

Let go of toxic relationships that are not elevating you or supporting your growth. Avoid negative people. This might be hard for you because family is one of our biggest stressors, and we feel compelled to tolerate more from family than we would from an external relationship. Many times, our familial interactions are obligatory, rather than an enjoyable gathering. Take a bird's-eye view of the relationship; zoom out as if you were watching it unfold for someone else. Would you ask for that dynamic, relationship, or interchange to come to a loved one? To you? If the answer is "No," then it might be time to make changes that are beneficial to your mental and emotional well-being. Surround yourself with positive people and with people you look up to, admire, and respect.

BEWARE OF TOXIC POSITIVITY

Know that everything is not perfectly perfect and that you don't have to be ecstatic each moment. All emotions have value and emotions are our teachers. Remember that most often everything is perfectly imperfect. We grow from the imperfections. We grow where there has been friction in our life, not from the status quo. You cannot appreciate a smoothly paved road, unless you have driven over a lot of potholes. The potholes and obstacles are the friction points that offer us a chance to appreciate the good things going on in our life. Can you smell that freshly paved tar?

LET GO OF A NON-NURTURING LIFESTYLE

Turn on your good genes with a positive mindset and healthy lifestyle choices. Recall our story of the twins and how their DNA was the same, yet their health was very different, based on their lifestyle choices.

BE AWARE OF YOUR BOUNDARIES

It is time to stop saying "Yes" when you don't want to. Be clear in your communications. "No thanks, that doesn't work for me" is a very empowering statement that honors your boundaries. You don't have to offer an explanation. When we really don't want to do something, but we do it out of obligation or for whatever reason, we can have a feeling of resentment. Resentment can turn to anger, and then we have lost the positive hormones, Law of Attraction, and our rest and digest mode, and instead have stressed ourselves and our hearts needlessly over something we could have said "No" to. Can you see how empowering and liberating the word "No" is? Notice this the next time you decline an invitation for something you do not want to participate in. Will your choice and answer be a "Divine Yes" or a "Sacred No?" What will saying "No" to allow space for you to say "Yes" to?

LISTEN TO YOUR GUT

It will tell you when things are not in your best interest. Your gut and your heart talk to each other. Is your heart listening to what your gut is telling you? We can have cognitive dissonance, a form of mental discomfort when we act with our heart and ignore our gut. We mentally change a belief when we have cognitive dissonance so that we can accept the choice versus feeling wrong about it. For example, a smoker might know that smoking causes cancer, but "just this one" releases him from feeling the conflict of knowing it is harmful behavior.

HAVE FAITH IN YOURSELF AND YOUR JOURNEY

You are here, doing the work. Your hard work and effort will not go unrewarded. What you put into your health will reap rewards. I encourage you to stay with your new healthier practices, even after your 66 days, and to keep showing up every day for yourself to show yourself and others that you care and that you matter.

LIVE YOUR LIFE WITH INTENTION

Live your life out loud and continue your great work as the driver of your car rather than passively riding along in the passenger seat every day. Showing up for yourself with intention means you have commitment for yourself, and this will increase your self-confidence.

BRING A BOOK OR YOUR JOURNAL WITH YOU EVERYWHERE

If you are stuck in a subway or bus or in a grocery line you can improve your mind or have an enjoyable and productive moment of self-enhancement. Take a look at my book recommendations on the "Bookshelf" in the "Resource Boutique" at the end of your book. Ditch TV, which can be a waste of time in shows with no value to your self-enhancement and expand your knowledge with books. Own this book and mark it up and highlight in it and make notes of areas you like, so you can reflect back on it when you flip through it. There is beauty in making a book yours. I highly suggest a visit to your library to check out books. You can save money, while enjoying the book. Please do not mark up a library book, though!

MEDITATE

Feel yourself vibrating energetically with positivity and a sense of possibility after meditation. Know how good this is for your mental and physical wellbeing. Steep in that good feeling of letting the outside world go, so you can tune-in to yourself. If you are having a moment of anxiety or stuck in traffic, pull out your tool of box-breathing and instead of getting frustrated at a delay, challenge yourself to see how chilled out you can emerge from the situation. I wish I had the box breathing tool when I was commuting home from work daily in Los Angeles years ago. My fifteen-mile commute sometimes took me three hours, and I usually did not arrive home in a chilled-out state!

TALK TO YOURSELF AS YOU WOULD TALK TO A LOVED ONE

We tend to be our own harshest critics. Notice negative self-talk and move to compassion for yourself. Look your accountability partner square in the eye in the bathroom mirror, and tell them how great they are! You are awesome!

DRINK PLENTY OF WATER

Ensure you are not dehydrated, which can lead to thicker, harder-to-pump blood for your heart. Take water with you in a glass water bottle to eliminate exposure to plastic. A rule of thumb is to have about (8) eight-ounce glasses of water a day.* Coffee is not water! When you drink coffee or any dehydrating caffeinated beverage, drink a glass of water with it to rehydrate.

*Check with your doctor about your daily hydration needs, especially if you are on fluid restrictions or are taking a diuretic medication.

WEAR BLUE LIGHT BLOCKING GLASSES WHEN USING YOUR COMPUTERS AND PHONES

Set your computer and phone on "night mode" to decrease disruption of your circadian rhythm. Circadian rhythm is the natural flow of wakefulness and sleep your body has in a 24-hour cycle, which can be disrupted by certain lighting.

ESTABLISH A SET ROUTINE FOR BEDTIME AND THE TIME YOU GET UP EACH DAY

Our body performs better with routine. When you get up, let in some natural morning light. These habits will help to set your innate natural circadian rhythm.

HAVE A HEALTHY SNACK WITH YOU AT ALL TIMES

Have a snack on-hand in case you feel low in energy or get detained for some reason. You can tuck a piece of fruit or a portable pack of nut butter in your bag or tote for an on-the-go snack.

ENSURE YOU ARE GETTING ENOUGH SLEEP

Rest when needed, especially if you have had a surgery or illness. It is easy to not know our new limitations after a surgery. Take it easy and do a little more each day, as your energy builds. Sleep is when our body restores itself. Avoid eating meals near bedtime. Ideally you want to have your bedtime at least a few hours after your dinner so your body can start the digestion process, and then can assume the restorative processes when you are sleeping. If your sleeping space isn't very dark, use an eye mask at night to help your body know it is nighttime. Earplugs are also a great tool to tune out any sounds.

CLEAR OUT YOUR LIVING SPACE

Clear the energy of your living space of unneeded and unwanted items to allow room for new things to come in. Consider donating items you do not want or need to an organization that can give things to people who really need them. Donate from a posture of purity of service to others, not in the interest of a tax write-off. Thank your items for serving you and wish them well on their way to help someone else.

ENSURE YOUR MUSIC IS UPLIFTING

What do the lyrics say? What is the beat? Is the singer a healthy and positive inspiration? Is the music calming to your nervous system and your heart?

MOVE IT!

To relieve stress, exercise, or even simply go for a mind-clearing walk. Consult with your doctor first about what exercise is best for you. If you feel inspired when listening to your music—move your body, as you listen to and heed any of its limitations.

COPE WITH STRESS

A sudden acute stressor such as a job loss or death of a loved one or even a beloved pet can cause the heart to be stunned. This condition, called "Broken Heart Syndrome," and medically known as "Takot-subo Cardiomyopathy," is a condition where the heart balloons up to look like an octopus's head, and can impair the hearts ability to pump. It is so important to get emotional support for your grief recovery. Get social support; call a friend or seek professional help if needed. Take a break from the stressor, if possible. Give yourself permission to grieve and then to step away from it. Chronic stress from grief releases hormones in our body that can lead to inflammation and hardening of the arteries.

COPE WITH DEPRESSION

This is very important. You may not even know you are depressed or that your mood and behavior is dimmed. I observed that a high percentage of my cardiac patients suffered from depression after their hospitalization and especially after their heart surgery. Patients seemed at a loss, and they really did not understand they were suffering from depression. Remember Abbie, from our earlier story? Abbie was very depressed in the hospital after her heart attack. After we discussed that she had her problem addressed, and she was safe, she was able to reframe her misfortune into an opportunity to think differently about her hospital stay. She shifted from "This happened to me, what am I going to do?" to "This happened to me, I am safe, I am supported, and I am going to get healthier because I am going to do X, Y and Z." Honor that this event happened to you, and know that you have the power to take control of the situation and create your own silver lining.

Please take a moment now to refer to the section of this book titled "Post-Op: Recovering From Your Heart Surgery." There, I have included a discussion about depression, which is applicable for everyone whether you have had surgery or not. Don't forget to return to me here after you check that out!

SMILE!

Smiling releases feel-good hormones into your body.

Do everyday activities that elevate your cardiac and overall health. (Do at your own pace, as you feel you can!)

BRUSH YOUR TEETH!

Brush your teeth at least twice daily. Floss after meals if you have enjoyed foods that stick in your teeth like corn on the cob. Floss before your last tooth brushing at night. Flossing first allows your toothbrush to help carry any loosened plaque of food particles away. Poor dental health can lead to bacterial infections which can cause inflammation in blood vessels and infections in the valves of the heart. See your dentist regularly every 6 months for checkups and cleanings. If you are out and about and cannot brush your teeth after eating, you can swish water in your mouth a few times to get out food particles and hydrate yourself at the same time.

TAKE THE "SHOELACE EXPRESS"

My beloved Uncle "Ritzie" would say this when he meant take a walk; he was going to take the "Shoelace Express." Take a walk instead of driving. Start a "Slush Fund" of money saved from not using car service or mass transit. Reward yourself periodically from your fund.

- Take the stairs instead of the elevator. Another option if there are lots of stairs is to get off of the elevator early and walk the remaining floors via the steps, as you are comfortably able. Start small and build up as you feel stronger and more comfortable.

- Park your car farther away from your destination. Walk to make up the distance.

- Get off the bus or subway or train a stop before your destination. Switch to the "Shoelace Express" and walk the rest of the way.

- Use a step monitor to check your daily walking step activity. Did you hit your goal today? You can record your wins and challenges in your journal.

RIDE A BIKE

Can you ride a bike instead of driving? A helmet and lights are recommended for your safety and may even be required by law in your town. Some cities have wonderful bike lanes and bikes you can rent for a day, if you do not have your own bike.

GROW YOUR OWN VEGGIES OR HERB GARDEN

Yes, you can even grow a plant on the windowsill. (An avocado pit counts!)

CONSIDER GETTING A DOG OR OTHER PET

Dogs offer companionship, keep you up and out on walks and you meet other people through our four-legged friends. Note: the commitment of owning a dog or any pet should be carefully considered, as this is a multiple year commitment with obligations of time, veterinary bills, food, and other costs. Consider if you will be leaving your pet alone for long periods of time. Being alone is okay for a cat, but not so much for a puppy, and what they could do to your couch when left unsupervised.

DEVOTE TIME TO PERSONAL GROWTH

Make time to enhance your mental, emotional, physical, and spiritual well-being. What passion projects would you like to pursue that will light you up? What book can you read that you won't want to put down because it speaks to you and you are getting so many takeaways? What class would you like to take? What certification and knowledge would you like to acquire? Take radical responsibility for your self-enhancement and get after it!

JOURNAL IT OUT

Whether you use a lined spiral bound notebook or a formal journal, it is great to write things down and reflect back on them. You can journal out anything that might be upsetting you, along with what you think you can do to help resolve it. You can journal all the good things happening for you, too. There are journals that have prompts, which offer you a thought to ponder as you write. Visit a bookstore or look online to find the different types and styles of journals that speak to you and inspire you. Write your thoughts authentically, from the heart and as if no one is looking.

PERFORM A RANDOM ACT OF KINDNESS

Help someone else. A good way to help yourself feel better is to help someone else feel better. Pay for the person behind you in line for coffee, leave a sticky note with a beautiful quote on it in a book in the library or somewhere in public for someone to find, do something special for your loved one, give a sincere compliment, smile at your waiter or cashier, ask how their day is going and stop to look them in the eye, hear them and listen to their answer. As humans, we all want to be honored, valued, seen, and heard.

CHECK IN WITH YOURSELF DAILY

Reflect during the daily chime time you set on your phone or clock with the phrase "How am I feeling right now?" Check in with your body, mind, heart, gut, and emotions. Many times, we blindly proceed into every minute instead of *thoughtfully* entering into it. Checking in with yourself before making a decision is a great way to observe

"How do I really feel about this?" Listening to your body, your gut, heart, and mind, and what they say to each other is key to understanding yourself.

CELEBRATE YOUR PROGRESS

As we approach the conclusion of our 66 days of *Heart to Soul Cardiac Wellness* together, if possible and if covered by your health insurance plan, see your doctor, get another set of labs drawn, and your vitals taken. When the lab results are available, document the data in the "End of Program" fields. Compare it to your original data. If you have been all-in and have done all the work, you should be feeling better and be seeing positive results, with the lab results to prove it! If you are unable to see your doctor right away, simply pause and notice how you are feeling at this juncture. Have you noticed a positive shift in your mindset? Do your clothes seem to fit better? Are you feeling a sparkle of vitality? How does your skin look? Has anyone commented that you "seem different?" Are you enjoying some new and different foods? If you are diabetic, are you seeing a nice trend downward in your morning glucose level on your graph? Has your doctor changed any of your medication dosages as a result of your health and lab trends? What does your accountability partner in the bathroom mirror think?

You are amazing! Great work! Keep on going! Remember to honor that good old friend "compassionate compliance" with yourself. I encourage you to continue your great work on your wellness, one bite at a time, one day at a time.

As you move forward, see your doctor regularly to monitor your labs, blood glucose, A1c, blood pressure, cholesterol, and weight. Continue to keep track of your values. Work together with your doctor to possibly decrease or even eliminate medications as your lab values trend positively and your feeling of wellness improves.

WEEKLY HOMEWORK
(CHECK OFF WHEN COMPLETED)

☐ As an exercise for you this next week, catch yourself every time you are thinking or saying anything negative. It may be surprising for you to observe and become aware of how much you focus on negativity and cynicism instead of what is going well in the moment. Replace the negative thought with a positive one. Instead of "Why am I sitting here in traffic waiting for this bulldozer to drive down the street?" this thoughtful moment can be switched to, "I have this extra time to listen to the radio and have some quiet time alone to reflect."

☐ Research "Sleep Hygiene" on www.sleepfoundation.org and implement the recommendations into your nightly routine.

☐ Complete your final journal assignments this week, reflecting on what you have learned from working with this book. What was your biggest takeaway? I would love to hear about your thoughts, struggles and successes. Please share them with me on my Instagram at @hearttosoulcw

☐ Share your new health knowledge with others. If we could all help each other out, think of how much better we could make the world! Please tell your friends and family about your book and encourage them to get their copy of *Heart to Soul Cardiac Wellness*, so they can get healthy too!

"ONE PERSON CAN MAKE A DIFFERENCE,
AND EVERYONE SHOULD TRY."

—JOHN F. KENNEDY, former President of the United States

Day 57: YOUR HEART TO SOUL DAILY JOURNAL

DATE: _____

DAILY WEIGHT:_____ A.M. GLUCOSE:_____

TODAY'S OVERALL FEELING OF WELLNESS:

1   2   3   4   5   6   7   8   9   10

INTENTION WORD FOR THE DAY:_____

TODAY I ACCOMPLISHED:

☐ Mindful breath work

☐ Mindful meditation (Duration _____)

☐ Joy & Meaning self-care activity:_____

3 THINGS I AM GRATEFUL FOR TODAY:

1.

2.

3.

WHAT'S ON YOUR MIND?

Day 58: YOUR HEART TO SOUL DAILY JOURNAL

DATE: _____

DAILY WEIGHT:_____   A.M. GLUCOSE:_____

TODAY'S OVERALL FEELING OF WELLNESS:

1   2   3   4   5   6   7   8   9   10

INTENTION WORD FOR THE DAY:_____

TODAY I ACCOMPLISHED:

☐ Mindful breath work

☐ Mindful meditation (Duration _____)

☐ Joy & Meaning self-care activity:_____

3 THINGS I AM GRATEFUL FOR TODAY:

1.

2.

3.

WHAT'S ON YOUR MIND?

Day 59: YOUR HEART TO SOUL DAILY JOURNAL

DATE: _____

DAILY WEIGHT: _____ A.M. GLUCOSE: _____

TODAY'S OVERALL FEELING OF WELLNESS:

1   2   3   4   5   6   7   8   9   10

INTENTION WORD FOR THE DAY: _____

TODAY I ACCOMPLISHED:

☐ Mindful breath work

☐ Mindful meditation (Duration _____)

☐ Joy & Meaning self-care activity: _____

3 THINGS I AM GRATEFUL FOR TODAY:

1.

2.

3.

WHAT'S ON YOUR MIND?

Day 60: **YOUR HEART TO SOUL DAILY JOURNAL**

DATE: _____

DAILY WEIGHT: _____ A.M. GLUCOSE: _____

TODAY'S OVERALL FEELING OF WELLNESS:

1   2   3   4   5   6   7   8   9   10

INTENTION WORD FOR THE DAY: _____

TODAY I ACCOMPLISHED:

☐ Mindful breath work

☐ Mindful meditation (Duration _____)

☐ Joy & Meaning self-care activity: _____

3 THINGS I AM GRATEFUL FOR TODAY:

1.

2.

3.

WHAT'S ON YOUR MIND?

Day 61: YOUR HEART TO SOUL DAILY JOURNAL

DATE: _____

DAILY WEIGHT: _____   A.M. GLUCOSE: _____

TODAY'S OVERALL FEELING OF WELLNESS:

1   2   3   4   5   6   7   8   9   10

INTENTION WORD FOR THE DAY: _____

TODAY I ACCOMPLISHED:

☐ Mindful breath work

☐ Mindful meditation (Duration _____)

☐ Joy & Meaning self-care activity: _____

3 THINGS I AM GRATEFUL FOR TODAY:

1.

2.

3.

WHAT'S ON YOUR MIND?

Day 62: YOUR HEART TO SOUL DAILY JOURNAL

DATE: _____

DAILY WEIGHT:_____   A.M. GLUCOSE:_____

TODAY'S OVERALL FEELING OF WELLNESS:

1   2   3   4   5   6   7   8   9   10

INTENTION WORD FOR THE DAY:_____

TODAY I ACCOMPLISHED:

☐ Mindful breath work

☐ Mindful meditation (Duration _____)

☐ Joy & Meaning self-care activity:_____

3 THINGS I AM GRATEFUL FOR TODAY:

1.

2.

3.

WHAT'S ON YOUR MIND?

Day 63: YOUR HEART TO SOUL DAILY JOURNAL

DATE: _____

DAILY WEIGHT: _____ A.M. GLUCOSE: _____

TODAY'S OVERALL FEELING OF WELLNESS:

1   2   3   4   5   6   7   8   9   10

INTENTION WORD FOR THE DAY: _____

TODAY I ACCOMPLISHED:

☐ Mindful breath work

☐ Mindful meditation (Duration _____)

☐ Joy & Meaning self-care activity: _____

3 THINGS I AM GRATEFUL FOR TODAY:

1.

2.

3.

WHAT'S ON YOUR MIND?

Day 64: **YOUR HEART TO SOUL DAILY JOURNAL**

DATE: _____

DAILY WEIGHT: _____ **A.M. GLUCOSE:** _____

TODAY'S OVERALL FEELING OF WELLNESS:

1 2 3 4 5 6 7 8 9 10

INTENTION WORD FOR THE DAY: _____

TODAY I ACCOMPLISHED:

- ☐ Mindful breath work
- ☐ Mindful meditation (Duration _____)
- ☐ Joy & Meaning self-care activity: _____

3 THINGS I AM GRATEFUL FOR TODAY:

1.

2.

3.

WHAT'S ON YOUR MIND?

Day 65: YOUR HEART TO SOUL DAILY JOURNAL

DATE: _____

DAILY WEIGHT:_____ A.M. GLUCOSE:_____

TODAY'S OVERALL FEELING OF WELLNESS:

1   2   3   4   5   6   7   8   9   10

INTENTION WORD FOR THE DAY:_____

TODAY I ACCOMPLISHED:

☐ Mindful breath work

☐ Mindful meditation (Duration _____)

☐ Joy & Meaning self-care activity:_____

3 THINGS I AM GRATEFUL FOR TODAY:

1.

2.

3.

WHAT'S ON YOUR MIND?

Day 66: **YOUR HEART TO SOUL DAILY JOURNAL**

DATE: _____

DAILY WEIGHT: _____ **A.M. GLUCOSE:** _____

TODAY'S OVERALL FEELING OF WELLNESS:

1   2   3   4   5   6   7   8   9   10

INTENTION WORD FOR THE DAY: _____

TODAY I ACCOMPLISHED:

☐ Mindful breath work

☐ Mindful meditation (Duration _____)

☐ Joy & Meaning self-care activity: _____

3 THINGS I AM GRATEFUL FOR TODAY:

1.

2.

3.

WHAT'S ON YOUR MIND?

YOU HAVE COMPLETED YOUR FIRST STEP ON YOUR HEALTH JOURNEY!

Congratulations! Well done!

"I DIDN'T COME THIS FAR, TO ONLY COME THIS FAR!"

—JESSE ITZLER, American entrepreneur, author, speaker, rapper

---

You did it! You have hopped into the wellness airplane and have accelerated down the runway, and now it's time for "Wheels up!" as you continue on your health journey—because it is a lifelong trip. This is the beginning of the new you. You are at the finish line of your 66-day plan, but you are also at a new starting line to move forward with the information you have learned. Pack your bags for the next part of this exciting trip!

I encourage you to share what you learn during your heart health journey with your friends and loved ones so they can become a part of your health team and they can get healthier, too. This 9 week plan is also wonderful to do together as a group, where you have additional support and camaraderie as you learn to make small changes with big impacts together. You can even buddy up and make it a health challenge for a friend in need of a lifestyle tune-up, or re-visit any or all of your weekly steps in the classes on www.hearttosoulcw.com.

> "OFTEN WHEN YOU THINK YOU'RE AT THE END OF SOMETHING, YOU'RE AT THE BEGINNING OF SOMETHING ELSE."
>
> **—FRED ROGERS, aka "Mr. Rogers"**

Together, focused on heart health, we can knock heart disease off the top spot as the leading cause of death in the U.S.

I hope you found the information in this book to be valuable, informative, and comforting on your journey to heart health. I love hearing about your stories of healing. I invite you to share your progress and how this book helped you in your review of my book on Amazon.com. Feel free to connect with me at www.hearttosoulcw.com, where you will also find additional resources to help you. Bright blessings to you on your journey to better health!

Thank you for allowing me the honor to be a part of your healing and wellness journey.

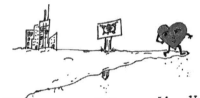

Following Your Heart is Frequently Scary... But Never Wrong

The Universe conspires with you to support you once you finally "jump." only the times when you step to the edge and hesitate is there confusion. Your heart leads you to the path less taken. The path of trusting your inner guidance to nudge you to keep showing up in full service. For some reason, each time we follow heart, it seems scary until you realize you are fully supported every single time.

— ♡ —

I cannot recall one single time, with an elevated view, that I was ever upset I followed my heart. You cannot be mistaken in service of your built-in GPS. There is a certain strange PULL and allurement that simply will not quit. Your heart is that bridge between your cosmic blueprint and the perfect unfolding here. Now.

Q: What are you standing on the precipice of? Go ahead...

3... 2... 1... ♥ Jump

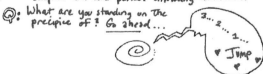

Used with permission from Yanik Silver, creator of the *Cosmic Journal*.

PART THREE

You've GOT THIS!

Pre-Op:
PREPARING FOR YOUR HEART SURGERY

Okay, you have been scheduled for a cardiac surgery. No matter what the surgery, it is daunting to think about. It can be scary to think about the unknown. Let's take a moment to breathe and to honor this time. Preparing yourself with knowledge and setting up your plan for recovery can ease your mind.

"FORTUNE FAVORS THE PREPARED MIND."

—LOUIS PASTEUR, French biologist, microbiologist, and chemist

---

Lots of people have sailed through the same surgery as you and are now living their lives vibrantly. Know you are not alone, and that you are supported here and you are ahead of the game because of your preparation with the information in this book. You have a plan. If you would like to either work one-on-one with me to prepare for or recuperate from your surgery, or you would like to take a group class with others for pre-op preparation or post-op recovery, please refer to my website www.hearttosoulcw.com for online class options.

LET'S GET YOU READY FOR SURGERY

First, we need to think about what is going to happen *after* surgery *before* you go into the hospital to help you adjust and have less stress as you transition back into your new life after surgery. Having a plan can help ease your mind.

Like a pilot when he or she enters into the cockpit to get the plane ready for its flight, it is important to have a checklist of things that will help you throughout your surgical experience. To follow is a list of things to set up before you have surgery, to help you while you are in the hospital, and to help make your recuperation at home smoother. Preparation is key. It might seem like a little extra effort now, but it will save you lots of time and aggravation later, when you really need to be focusing on your recovery. It is very helpful to share Part Three of this book with your spouse/partner/caregiver/loved ones, so they understand the scope of what is happening behind the scenes, and they can prepare themselves, too!

☐ **Prepare Your Directives.**

I want to take a moment here to advise that it is always—not only now, before a surgery, but at all times—important to have your will and financial paperwork in order. Having these documents sorted out will ensure that you and your family are at ease, and there are clear instructions for direction in your medical care and your financial management. Show your family where all the paperwork is. Have your health proxy paperwork (stating who will speak for you in the event you cannot answer questions, i.e. if during your operation, input is needed on the course of surgical direction for the surgeons) and advanced directives (living will information, durable power of attorney, DNR—Do Not Resuscitate order, organ donor information) paperwork available for your family to have on hand when you have surgery.

☐ **Set up communications for updates on your status.**

Set up, or have a family member set up, a communication portal such as a phone contact list or a page on Facebook, an email list, a standing Zoom update call or Instagram account update to let everyone know your progress, instead of everyone calling each other but not getting accurate or updated information. Taking control of the information process eliminates family members from getting a constant stream of requests for information. Make one person the contact person for the family, but the designated communication site, such as those listed above, is to be checked first before calling that contact person. You can make a statement on your site such as "While we greatly appreciate your support, we ask that you refrain from calling or texting us and instead please view the following page for updates, so that we can spend uninterrupted time with our loved one."

On your info page, let folks know you will give the go-ahead when they can call or come to visit you in the hospital. Tell them not to bring flowers. They are not allowed in the hospital and can make a patient sick. Tell them not to bring gifts as it will be something else you will have to transport home when you are discharged from the hospital. All of that can wait until you can receive them at home. The gift of their presence is the gift! Refrain from extra visitors the first few days though, until you get acclimated to your post-op conditions. This will allow you time to rest, while you also gradually get off pain medications.

☐ **Make arrangements for one different person each day to bring food to your family members at home while you are away in the hospital.**

Not having to shop and cook and clean helps relieve stress and burden on the family members who are concentrating on you. People really *do* want to help you out, and this gives them something to do. You may want to assign this meal preparation task to your friends who are super great cooks. (Wink!) Make sure you make them aware of any food allergies or nutrition plans.

☐ **Make arrangements for caregivers for any young children at home while you are away in the hospital.**

☐ **Make a "Wing-Person" chart to give to your point person and the people on the chart.**

Arrange for a few key people, one at a time, to be stationed bedside as soon as you are able to have visitors in the hospital. This is *not* so they will occupy your time or energy in communication; *they are there to support your needs.* They are there if you have pain, need repositioning or need water, to charge your phone, take notes for you and help you with anything that can help your immediate non-medical needs. They can help you if you are confused after surgery, which is very common. They are there if you want them to be, to provide a feeling of comfort and security. This rotating "Wing-Person" can also call your nurse if needed.

☐ **Get your hair cut prior to surgery.**

Let your beard, legs, and armpits go for now and until you are home from the hospital. Shaving can cause micro cuts, which could be a potential source of infection. There will be plenty of time for re-beautification once you are home.

☐ **Do not wear nail polish or gel manicures to the hospital.**

Your nailbeds need to be free of blockages and in their natural state so your oxygenation can be monitored.

☐ **Leave all jewelry at home.**

Earrings, necklaces, and bracelets may be easily lost as they fall out into bedsheets, which are changed frequently. Rings can cut off circulation in your finger if your hand gets swollen after surgery.

☐ **Load a special playlist for healing onto your phone.**

You may want to incorporate some of the following to try, and they are best enjoyed with headphones or earbuds to maximize the sound experience.

- Save some **guided meditations** into an email file. There are lots of guided meditation options online, and I have listed some apps in the "Resource Boutique" at the end of your book.

- Download singing bowl **Sound Healing** which incorporates the sound vibration of crystal bowls, when struck, or played. Singing bowls in particular are tuned to a frequency matching our energy centers, called "Chakras" in the body. Many times we experience and hold emotions and wounds in our tissues—think of the knots you can get in your shoulders when stressed. Sound healing helps to release the energy from these "knots" of physical and mental emotion that have translated to our tissues. Singing bowl sound healing may help clear some of that stored energy, which in turn may help to release the physical holding and pain. You can meditate while listening to sound healing. Sound healing facilitates meditation because it can put your brain in a more relaxed state.

- Download **Solfeggio healing energy deep Hertz** music.

- Download **Binaural Beats** music. Depending on the Hertz frequency, Binaural beat frequencies are linked to relaxation, sleep, anxiety reduction, meditation, happiness, creativity, concentration, and alertness. Experiment listening to the many free Binaural Beat frequencies online and how you feel and respond to them.

- Download healing **Gong** sounds. Gong sounds have healing energetic soundwaves that literally get your body cells vibrating when you hear and feel the music in person. Listening online is almost like being there!

- Download your **favorite podcast's** current episodes so they are ready to go.

☐ **Create a little inspirational vision board to take to the hospital.**

You can get your family or kids involved in this project, or even completely give ownership to them as this gets them involved in being a part of your healing process. This vision board will be for your happiness wall in the hospital and then at home. A client of mine created a vision board of all the things she was going to do after she recuperated. She had pictures of her dog on his leash, her chair and towel set up at the beach, knitting needles and a ball of yarn, a cookbook and a picnic table. She also had a few pictures of her family at celebrations.

☐ **Prepare your sleep space for your return.**

Create a new area of special healing talismans, crystals and things you love that will be there to welcome you home. Do any special nesting or sprucing up in your space so you have it nice, clean, and organized when you come home.

☐ **Have everything you need bedside (for at home and in the hospital) within reach and in a plastic washable tub.**

Organizing things and containing your bedside items will eliminate things falling over or get knocked to the floor, where they can become a tripping hazard. Have the tub ready for you, post-op. **Stock it up** with all of your comfort items like lip balm, tissues, wipes, the TV remote, a book, phone, charger, water bottle, hand lotion, eyeglasses, etc. Your throat may be sore after surgery, and a throat spray is preferable over lozenges, as a lozenge is a choking hazard if you are lying in bed. Have a trash bag or trash can handy for used tissues and wipes. To follow in this chapter is a checklist of things to bring to the hospital bedside and you can use this checklist for your home bedside as well.

☐ **Optimize your lungs.**

Prior to surgery, it is a great idea to optimize the oral and nasal cavities to be prophylactic (taking measures to prevent disease) against infection and pneumonia. Sitting up in a chair as much as possible is preferable to lying in bed to help your lungs fully expand.

☐ **Belly breaths/deep breathing.**

We want to focus on expanding from the belly on up to the entire lung cavity, before and after surgery to keep the little air sacks at the lung bases called "alveoli" open. This helps to prevent a lung infection. You should be positioned upright as much as possible when in bed post-op, facilitating deep breathing. Deep belly breaths help with pressing on the diaphragm, which passively presses the intestines and lymph, our cleansing and drainage fluid system, which helps to circulate blood and nutrients. You can start practicing these deep belly breaths pre-op, so you will be accustomed to performing them for your post-op recovery.

> **PRO TIP**: Shower with a few drops of eucalyptus oil splashed into the shower for a spa-like moment while having the benefits of the aromatherapy and antibacterial power from its essence. Enjoy a belly breath or two while in the shower. Heck, enjoy a belly breath or two anywhere!

☐ Incentive spirometer.

An incentive spirometer is a device to help you inhale and hold your breath briefly to expand and exercise your lungs to prevent pneumonia post-op. You may be able to order one from a drug store or surgical supply store prior to surgery. The goal is to do ten repetitions per hour post-op. Avoid hyperventilation, by taking the breaths slowly. Take your time; nice and easy does it. Give it a try pre-op so you are comfortable with this as part of your recovery post-op.

> **PRO TIP**: In the hospital, ask the nurses for alcohol wipes, and you may want to buy your own for your hospital toolkit, to wipe off your incentive spirometer mouthpiece after each use.

☐ Gargle.

Gargle daily with a mouthwash that contains colloidal silver, a bacteriostat which guards against bacterial growth.

☐ Manuka honey.

The higher the Kfactor (pollen level), the better. Honey is bacteriostatic, meaning that it protects against bacteria. Have a teaspoon a day (if non-diabetic), and put this in your hospital toolkit with disposable (biodegradable) spoons. Manuka honey can be expensive, so reserve this honey for medicinal use only, not for use with your cooking, coffee, or tea.

☐ Optimize your blood.

Eat and cook with the following: garlic, onions, and iron rich foods-like spinach, tofu, broccoli, and quinoa.

> **ALERT!** Important Note: Please check with your physician if you are on blood thinners due to the blood thinning effects of garlic and leafy greens.

☐ Cook with anti-inflammatory foods.

Add grated ginger to foods, or in water for tea. Sprinkle turmeric onto your food, but you must add black pepper to it to make it more easily absorbable for your body. Eliminate sugar and processed white flour product baked goods. As much as possible, eat clean, nutritious foods. The goal is to put the best ingredients into your body to help it heal.

LET'S TAKE A LOOK AT OUR DAILY ACTIONS

Mandatory homework assignment: If you are at home, pre-op, make your activities flow today as if you ARE post-op.

UPPER CABINETS

Will you be able to reach up to the upper cabinets to get canned foods rice, cups or plates down? Move all things from an upper level which requires you to reach, down to the countertop level. This may make your house feel cluttered, but it will be helpful for you to have your things within reach.

OPEN JARS IN ADVANCE

You won't be able to open jars right away, so the day before you come home, have a family member or designee open any jars of food you have pre-designated and bottle caps loosened, with a reminder note placed on the refrigerator that you are all set and the caps are loosened. Will you be able to move the large water filter pitcher? Not right away, so fill smaller bottles for hydration for when you come home.

Make sure all toiletries, supplies and food you need are stocked up prior to surgery.

ANTICIPATE YOUR PHYSICAL CAPABILITIES AND NEEDS

Will you be able to pull open a glass sliding door to the patio? No, not at first. Will you be able to slide open the medicine cabinet? Not at first, so you may have to reorganize your things, move them down to a reachable area, and leave the medicine cabinet open on your side if possible for access.

> **Note:** Your doctor will give you a list of activities you should avoid. Listen to your body, too. If you do not feel good or start to have pain doing something, back off. If you have any palpitations or arrhythmias, chest pain, or you do not feel right, as always, follow your doctor's instructions, call your doctor, or call 9-1-1.

LET'S TALK ABOUT POOP

No one wants to talk about poop, but we need to. Think about what is going to happen in the hospital if you have a steak or huge bulky constipating meals before you go into the hospital. We want "smooth sailing" for your poops when you are in the hospital! Try to eat clean, light foods with lots of fiber that will help you to evacuate your bowels prior to going into the hospital. You want to set yourself up for easy poops in the hospital. It will be easier on you, your heart, the other patients and the hospital staff.

> **A word about pain meds:** Certain pain medications can make you constipated. We want to avoid constipation, as we do not want to push down during a bowel movement, which can impact the heart. The doctor may put you on a bowel regimen which is a

combination of medications to facilitate bowel movements during your stay in the hospital. Check with your doctor, and if potassium is not an issue, ask your doctor if you can drink prune juice or eat dried prunes or dates to help along your bowels.

PLAN FUTURE EVENTS

Plan some fun activities for after you have recuperated for a bit of time, so you have those outings to look forward to. Mark them on your calendar.

MAKE YOUR SENDOFF A CELEBRATION!

Have a gathering/prayer circle/launch/pep-rally a day or two before surgery, to have a super supportive sendoff with friends and family. You can share the communication portal you have set up so people can check in on your progress. Enjoy being celebrated!

When you go to the hospital, give your dentures, eyeglasses, hearing aids, cane, wheelchair, scooter, walker, and any other health aids to your family member, or to the intake nurse or staff for storage. Do not wear any jewelry to the hospital.

PRE-OP APPOINTMENT

CONSENT FORM

The consent form presents the risks (and benefits) of surgery presented by a doctor to you in a worst-case scenario. Remember that you possibly had the same ultimate risk for a prior cardiac assessment or procedure such as a cardiac catheterization. You are in the hands of a fine surgeon, who has spent years in training doing your surgery. You have worked hard to fully optimize your body in preparation for this. Your baseline health going into your surgery is amplified and uplifted due to your preparation.

You may sign a HIPAA (Health Insurance Portability and Accountability Act) form which ensures that your healthcare information is private and protected by law.

You may have the following and other tests:

- Blood work
- Urine test
- Electrocardiogram (EKG)
- Echocardiogram (ECHO)
- Chest x-ray

ALLERGIC REACTIONS

Let all medical staff know what allergies you have, what medications you are on, the dosage, and how frequently you take them.

DRUG INTERACTIONS

If you are on an anticoagulant (blood thinner), let the doctors and nurses know. Some medicines need to be stopped or changed to a different one before surgery.

INSURANCE COVERAGE

IMPORTANT! Double check with the surgery scheduler to ensure all your doctors are in your insurance network, so there are no surprises of additional charges or bills. Ensure all pre-op authorization if applicable, is completed and approved by insurance.

> **PRO TIP:** Ask for an itemized bill at the end of your stay so that you can verify you were not erroneously charged.

SOME HELPFUL RESOURCES FOR YOU

- www.keepmyrx.org
- www.allianceforpatientaccess.org
- www.patientadvocate.org
- www.naic.org
- www.hhs.gov/regulations/complaints-and-appeals/index.html
- www.cms.gov/CCIIO
- www.askebsa.dol.gov or (866) 444-3272

CARDIAC REHABILITATION

Are you a candidate for cardiac rehab? Cardiac rehab programs provide a supervised and monitored exercise program specific for cardiac patients, which is very important in the recovery process. Does your health insurance cover cardiac rehab? It might be a good idea to check into that. Cardiac rehab can not only help your physical recovery, it can help your mental and emotional recovery as well. It is a nice transition from hospital to home, and can step you into a recovery regimen with others who have had a similar experience. You might even make a new friend group of other Cardiac Thrivers there!

VISITING NURSE

Will you be eligible for a visiting nurse when you are first discharged, especially if you do not go to cardiac rehab or if you live alone and do not have family to help you? Will your insurance cover a visiting nurse?

SUPPORT GROUP

What groups would you like to join so you will have some supportive camaraderie? Are there blog posts you can read post-op? Support groups are great to research before you go in for your surgery. Be mindful not to go too far down the rabbit hole though on looking at these sites now, because you are not there in your recuperation yet and you could get way ahead of yourself and start focusing on things that will not pertain to your recovery. Can your doctor recommend some local support groups? Does your doctor or medical facility have a buddy program for someone you can contact to help step you through any questions or concerns you have?

PRE-OP MORNING

> **Most important reminder:**
>
> **DO NOT HAVE ANYTHING TO EAT OR DRINK
> AFTER MIDNIGHT BEFORE YOUR SURGERY.**
>
> **Note: Check with your doctor-these are standard pre-op directives; however, you may have instructions specifically tailored to your needs.** The reason why you are not to eat or drink anything is so that your stomach will be empty and you will not vomit during surgery. This would create unnecessary complications and could result in aspiration pneumonia.

GET PSYCHED UP!

Set the alarm for a few minutes early so you have time to mentally prepare, center and ground yourself, meditate to set a tone for success, and to honor your body and your journey. Take some long, slow, deep belly breaths. Breathe in to the count of four slowly, breathe out to the count of seven, puffing your belly out as you inhale, drawing it in as you exhale. Give thanks for the opportunity to have this option for surgery and for the medical team helping you and your support team cheering for you.

OPTIMIZE YOUR ORAL CARE THE MORNING OF SURGERY.

Brush your teeth well, and gargle with salt water to moisten your mucous membranes since you have not been drinking.

FACE THE FEAR

Fear is our greatest obstacle in all things in life, and can prevent us from moving forward. Once we dive in to whatever it is we must tackle, we are through the fear and not in that moment any longer. On this morning, the day of your surgery, let's shift from fear to feelings of gratitude, for the surgeon and their team, for the wonderful support you have, and for the health and vitality you are bringing to the path of your recovery. Shifting to gratitude will help control and tamp down that fear. It's pretty difficult to feel two emotions at once. Practice deep belly breathing as you remember:

"THE COMEBACK IS ALWAYS STRONGER THAN THE SETBACK."
—UNKNOWN

ARM YOURSELF WITH THESE POWERFUL AFFIRMATIONS:

- I am healthy.
- I am supported.
- I am safe.
- I am grounded.

- I am loved.

- I've got this.

- I release fear.

- I am ready, and watch out because I am going to come back stronger than ever!

THINGS FOR YOUR FAMILY TO ASK WHEN YOU ARRIVE AT THE HOSPITAL FOR SURGERY

- What time will the surgery be? Unless this is the first case, this is an *approximate* time. There may be a case ahead of you, which may run into extra time, then the room needs to be cleaned and prepared for you.

- How long will the surgery be? Remember these are *approximations*.

- Where can we wait while the surgery is being performed?

- Will we be able to get any updates during the operation?

- When and where and how often can we visit after surgery?

Reminder: After hospital check-in, family should take home your jewelry, medications, eyeglasses, dentures, hearing aids, hairpins, hairpieces, underwear, contact lenses, prosthetics, canes, walking assist devices, wallet, and anything else you brought with you. You may not be returning to the same area as you were pre-op. Ask where you will be received post-op, and what the process is as you get better, and where you will be moved after that. Some hospitals are set up for recuperation in the same room, and some hospitals have special units or rooms for just out of the operating room, to intensive care, to step down, to cardiac rehab, or home.

The following is a list of items to have at the hospital for your recovery. Have someone bring them to you a day or so post-op, as there may not be adequate storage space in the hospital for your personal effects.

TO BRING TO THE HOSPITAL CHECKLIST:

- ☐ Sweater, sweatshirt or shawl to drape over your shoulders initially, then graduate to a robe. At first you may have trouble reaching around to put your arms into a robe, so maybe get a size up to make it easier to put on. Ensure it is not too long and that the belt is inside the belt loops as the belt could possibly be a tripping hazard.
- ☐ Slip-resistant socks or slippers
- ☐ Toothbrush and toothpaste
- ☐ Dry shampoo
- ☐ Deodorant
- ☐ Hairbrush
- ☐ Hand lotion (for hands only)
- ☐ Facial care products

- ☐ Lip balm
- ☐ Hand sanitizer
- ☐ Non-scented wipes
- ☐ Your own universal remote for the TV
- ☐ Soft tissues
- ☐ Reading materials
- ☐ Your journal and pens
- ☐ Sketchbook and coloring pencils
- ☐ Prunes and dates, if approved by your doctor
- ☐ Bottles of water
- ☐ Your phone, earbuds, and phone charger
- ☐ U shaped neck pillow for neck support
- ☐ A bin or container to keep all this contained at your bedside so items don't roll around out of reach or accidently get knocked to the floor.
- ☐ A notepad and pens to keep a list of questions prepared and for note taking
- ☐ For female post-op open-heart patients, you will need a bra to wear 24 hours a day for 6 weeks, unless otherwise noted by your physician. Get one without underwire, that you will be able to get in and out of easily. Check with your doctor to see if they have any recommendations of the type of bra that would be best for you. You may want to get a couple of different sized ones in case you are swollen after surgery.

- [ ] Essential oils (IF YOU ARE IN A PRIVATE ROOM). Use lavender for sleep, at nighttime, and a citrus for alertness in the daytime. You can put a drop or two of essential oil directly on your bedsheets to get their uplifting aromatherapy benefit. Try them out at home to make sure they are calming and agree with you before you take them to the hospital. Brands I use for their therapeutic quality may be found in the "Boutique" section of my website, www.hearttosoulcw.com.

- [ ] Your going home outfit, including slip-on loafer-like shoes that are easy to get on, and a coat and hat if it is winter.

- [ ] Pack a crystal or rock or shell to take with you to have in your hospital room to serve as your Earth friend and accompaniment to symbolize all the love and support you have from the Universe.

> **Note:** Because your slippers and products will have been in the hospital, I recommend using trial sizes and inexpensive articles and discarding your products when you leave the hospital. The fewer things that touch the hospital and that you bring into your home, the better. If you bring an article home, wipe it down with disinfectant wipes when you get home. Wash any clothing you have worn or have brought home immediately.

LET'S TALK ABOUT WHAT ELSE YOU CAN EXPECT

If you are already in the hospital or are checking-in to the hospital, you will have a pre-op check-in by a nurse, and you may have to sign any final paperwork.

You will also be consented by an anesthesiologist. This is a very key member of your medical team, and a person who is often overlooked until you enter the operating room. It is nice to meet your anesthesiologist team member in advance of your surgery, if possible. They will be the ones putting and keeping you asleep, pain free and comfortable during your procedure. They will be your wing person by your head in the operating room.

Please refrain from smoking, especially immediately prior to your surgery. This will clamp down and constrict the very arteries the doctor may need to work on in surgery.

When you go into the operating room, gather the medical team for a moment to have a huddle with you. Express your gratitude and thank them in advance. This is a moment to help them step back, recalibrate and to see you as "their person" rather than as "a case." It establishes a connection between you and them for this very intimate time you will be sharing together.

> **Remember your new credo:**
>
> **"The comeback is always stronger than the setback!"**

Know that you have done as much thoughtful prep work and health optimization as possible in your timeframe, so you are set up for success!

> **Your mantra for rolling into the operating room is:**
>
> **"I am safe and I am supported."**

WHILE YOU ARE IN THE HOSPITAL AND FOR YOUR POST-OP RECOVERY:

- Let the nurse know how to reach your family, so he or she can record it in your bedside nurse chart (if the hospital has one), and in your electronic medical record chart.

- Let the nurses and doctors know who your health proxy is.

- Notify your nurses and doctors of allergies, especially to seafood.

- Let your doctors and nurses know about vision, dental or hearing health issues so they are aware. Example; if you are hard of hearing and use a hearing aid, the staff needs to know, so they can speak louder for you.

- Give the doctors and nurses the name and contact information of your primary medical provider.

Please do keep in mind to cluster all nursing requests to honor their professional time, knowing that they have other patients like you to care for, too. The same goes for questions for the nurse or doctor. Take a pad and pen to the hospital to write down your questions to ask at one time. Write down their responses, because it is easy to forget, as there is so much going on, and you will have frequent interruptions in the hospital.

It is extremely important to have a person with you for your in-hospital bedside rounds or for your pre-op and post-op doctors' appointments as a note taker when your doctor is giving you information and when you have questions to ask. The note taker can concentrate on recording the answers while you assimilate information the doctor is telling you. It can be overwhelming to try to listen and take notes at the same time. The note taker is a key assignment for your "Wing-Person" while you are in the hospital as well.

- Ask how the call bell works and ensure it is always within your reach.

- Ask how your bed or special chair works.

- Ask where the bathroom is and how it works.

- Ask how to use the room phone and TV. Is there a charge?

- Ask what the visiting hours are.

- Ask if someone can stay the nights with you in your room. Some facilities offer 24/7 visiting hours and provide a cot for a loved one or visitor to sleep on. Sometimes a visitor is allowed to stay overnight, but they may have to rough it in a chair. Keep in mind this "Wing-Person" will need to bring in their own toiletries.

FOR YOU AND YOUR CAREGIVERS TO READ

After your operation, you may have a tube in your mouth for breathing assistance and many types of intravenous and centrally placed lines in you and drains coming out of your body. The good news is that you will be sedated. While the operation may just be over, the medical team needs to get you all set up in your post-op recovery area. Family will need to wait a little longer to see you, until you are all settled in, and this additional time for the staff needs to be honored so they can do so, safely and without interruption.

When you begin waking up, you may hear beeps and bubbling and alarms. These are all routine sounds of the equipment around you. Do not try to pull on anything. Do not touch your wound or bandages or pull on any tubing. Know that in time, and as your body is ready, you will be taken off these machines. The ventilator tube in your mouth may feel uncomfortable, and you will be taken off of this as soon as possible. The medical team wants to get you off this equipment, too.

When family and visitors are allowed to come in, **THEY FIRST NEED TO WASH THEIR HANDS EXTREMELY WELL— AND THIS GOES FOR EVERY VISIT!** They also need to wash their hands well upon leaving.

> **Note:** Additional hygiene and safety measures may be employed during and after the COVID-19 pandemic.

You will not look your usual beautiful self after the operation. You will be pale and swollen because your body is not and has not been in full circulation mode as if you were up and about, walking around. Your temperature may be cool. You may have a tube coming out of your mouth, attached to a ventilator to help you breathe. You were sedated and will still be, so you will not be responding for a little while. The beauty of these sedations is they usually cause amnesia so you probably won't remember any part of this event. You will have machines and monitors recording measurements of your cardiac and respiratory functions. You will not be in pain. You will have intravenous drugs to support your heart, for sedation, for pain, possibly for glucose control, possibly antibiotics, electrolyte replacement and for hydration. You will have a Foley catheter placed into your urethra to your bladder, to measure your urine output. You will have central lines placed and an arterial line to measure blood pressure internally, to take necessary blood samples without constantly poking you. You may have chest tubes and drains to help drain off excess fluids. All of this is standard procedure, and one by one they will be removed as your body is ready. Each day will bring a shedding of more things, because after all, you can't go home with all that equipment attached to you!

It is important for you as a family and your caregivers to know this information so you can be prepared, at least in your mind that you will see a different loved one, temporarily. It can be frightening for you to see your special person with all of these devices and monitors, but rest assured all of this is how the medical and surgical teams routinely support a patient through the post-op recovery process.

FOR BEDSIDE VISITORS: WHAT TO DO POST-OP

This is a new event for your loved ones and visitors to experience, too. To follow is a guide to share with visitors and caregivers, about what you can expect during the post-op experience in your role as a visitor, and how you can best support your special person.

It is important to let your loved one know that the operation is over, explain to them what is going on, and help them to remain calm. Due to sedation and having possibly been on a bypass machine, they will require frequent re-orienting to situation, place, and time. Five minutes after you tell them what is going on, you may see a crinkle in their brow and again, note confusion and again need to inform them that the operation is over and they are OK. Keep them from pulling any tubing; sit bedside and holding their hand if need be. Keep it simple to start. Continue to reorient them and let them know they are safe. Talk to them about other things also; like what's going on with their favorite TV show or team. Give them a daily update on family members, events, sports, the dog or cat, the neighbors, friends and anything they have an interest in and follow.

Your role as family members and supportive visitors is to be bedside cheerleaders. Even when your person is on sedation, they can feel your support and presence. They likely won't remember what you are telling them, but they will be aware of your presence in the moment. Patients may have delirium from being woken repeatedly for EKG, Echocardiogram, X-Ray, bloodwork and medications. This is also why ongoing reorientation for the patient and a bedside presence is important. Some families come and leave in a large group. This can be taxing on a patient energetically and makes it difficult to work in the room if you are a nurse. I recommend instead that one person at a time visit, and this way, the patient has someone bedside if they need help. Again, this is for your support, not to drain your energy from social visits.

Whatever your family can do to support you is a positive step for your recovery. Because there likely will not be windows where you are initially recuperating, it is important for family to tell you what day and date and time of day it is. Some of those hospital rooms can be as confusing as a Las Vegas casino, and it is helpful when family can help orient you.

Playing your favorite calming music on low volume is great, and prayers are inspiring.

> **Do not give any food or liquids to the patients, ESPECIALLY if the patient is still on a ventilator.**

They may signal they want water, and boy can they be persistent, but do *not* give it to them. This could cause them to vomit with the breathing tube in their lungs and result in an aspiration pneumonia. The nursing staff will periodically clean and moisten their mouth and keep them comfortable until the patient is extubated (they are taken off the ventilator).

(Don't worry-you as the patient will be given ice chips, then liquids after you have been taken off the ventilator, and then gradually advanced to solid foods.)

Cheer your loved one on: "Great! You are off the ventilator!" After they are extubated, (taken off the ventilator) they will get the go ahead for ice chips. "Let's focus on the breathing and having an ice chip!" Emotional support is critical to helping recovery. Little wins matter and are a cause for celebration! Their voice may be raspy at first due to the tube that was in their windpipe (trachea), and their throat may be a bit sore. Ice chips will help soothe the throat. Do not give the patient throat lozenges, as lozenges and sucking candies are a choking risk. If there are any meal concerns or food allergy concerns, let the nurses and doctors know. For example, if you want a vegan, kosher or halal meal or are allergic to shellfish, let the nurses and doctors know so your meal requirements can be met. Food will be advanced slowly from puree to solids, once you get the go ahead you can eat.

FIRST VISITS WILL BE BRIEF

Based on the hospital's visitor policy, you may be able to have someone bedside with you around the clock, as noted prior, for support, not socialization. As a nurse, I welcomed the help the patient received from a family member or friend bedside. I liked that the patient had a "Wing-Person" at their bedside.

PLEASE NOTE

Just as you would not want to be interrupted every five minutes at work with a question, the nurses and medical staff are doing work and they have other patients and their needs in addition to you and yours. It is very helpful to your medical team if you cluster all your questions and needs for them and request them all at one time as much as possible, when they can give you attention to address your needs. Bring a notepad and pen with you so you can make a list of questions for the nurses and doctors, and write down the answers. Respect that the nursing staff are under a lot of pressure to get things accomplished for your family member in a timely manner. A "Thank You!" to your doctors and nurses and caregivers goes a long way and is so appreciated. They are working very hard for you!

DO NOT FEEL BAD ABOUT TELLING PEOPLE AT ANY TIME THAT YOU DO NOT WANT VISITORS

This is your time to use your energy for healing. It may drain you if you feel you have to be "up" to socialize.

RECEIVING ASSISTANCE

As much as they would like, family can be involved in your activities of daily living, such as helping you brush your hair, using the bathroom and walking. Always check with the nurse first about what you can help with and what the patient is approved to do and with whose assistance. This will help everyone feel more comfortable.

REMEMBER THAT IT IS GOOD TO STAY ON TOP OF YOUR PAIN

Do not wait until you are really in a lot of pain to ask for a medication. If you haven't had your pain meds in a while, and you anticipate getting up for a big walk, ensure you have your pain meds before you start the walking, so it will be more comfortable for you. If you don't need the meds, even better. As you heal and get stronger, you will need pain medications less.

When sitting on the edge of the bed with your legs over the side before you get up to walk, make sure you do not feel dizzy.

If you feel dizzy, let your nurse know and wait until you do not feel dizzy. Do *not* cross your legs as this negatively impacts your circulation. You will most likely also have on SCDs (Sequential Compression Devices), that are like inflatable massagers on your lower legs to help facilitate circulation. Make sure these are detached from your legs before you attempt to walk, so you do not risk falling. Always use your call bell to ask for assistance, especially in the beginning. You will eventually become more autonomous. At first a few steps from the bed to a chair will be a huge win. You may have an assortment of IVs, monitoring lines and chest tubes to start, so take it easy and be open to assistance.

> Allow yourself the gift of time, and patience.

PREPARING FOR DISCHARGE

As the medical team is preparing you for discharge, **double check with the team that your prescriptions have been sent to your pharmacy.** You may want a family member to call to check pharmacy hours and to verify your prescription is ready. Make sure that you know and clearly understand what medications you are taking, why you are taking them, and their dosage and frequency. Make a copy of your discharge medication list to keep in your wallet for readiness in the event you see other doctors, as they will need to know what your medications are. Give a copy to your doctors. Ensure your family has a copy of this medication list as well, and update it and redistribute it as your medications change.

Post-Op:
RECOVERING FROM YOUR HEART SURGERY

Whew! You are discharged! You get to go HOME! If you are reading this chapter because you have just completed your surgery, after you have finished all of Part Three of this book, start at the beginning of *Heart to Soul Cardiac Wellness* to kick off your wellness journey. You have the tools right here in your hands to help you travel a new path to heart health.

> Please read the prior chapter regarding pre-op preparation, as it has some information that you can still put into play for your recovery, such as how to set up your home in preparation for your post-op needs.

You will have prescriptions for medications and a medical plan from your doctor, and this book will serve as your "prescription for your plan for heart health and and overall wellness." Use this book daily and with mindfulness. Following Jesse Itzler's coaching advice from *Build Your Life Resume*: "No Zero Days." We are going to make every day count as you move forward dedicated to living healthfully, body, mind, and *Heart to Soul*.

LET'S TALK ABOUT WHAT YOU CAN DO AND EXPECT WHEN YOU GET THE GREEN LIGHT TO GO HOME

Put all of your your doctors' office numbers in your phone so they are readily available if needed.

GET YOUR MEDICATIONS ON THE WAY HOME

When you call the pharmacy before you leave the hospital to make sure your meds are ready, give the pharmacist a heads up that you are coming directly from the hospital so they will be ready by the time you arrive. Get a pill box at the pharmacy so you can arrange Monday through Sunday, breakfast, lunch, and dinner time meds. If you don't have a bathroom scale, pick one up if you can while you are at the pharmacy. Know when you are taking each medication, why, and any side-effects you can anticipate. If you are on a blood thinner, ask what side effects and special care instructions you will need to follow.*

*Important note: You may have food considerations due to your medications which will supersede any nutritional information in the previous chapters.

YOU WILL NEED TO BUILD UP YOUR STRENGTH, SO BE GENTLE WITH YOURSELF

The first time doing anything will be new, and you will get tired easily, as you have decreased energy reserve and have not been moving around for a while.

ESTABLISH A ROUTINE

When you wake up in the morning, use the bathroom, weigh yourself, drink a little water, meditate, and have breakfast. Next up, take a little walk, increasing the amount of time every day, then a rest. Set up goals for yourself to accomplish each day. Log your progress in your 66 daily journal pages in this book. You can use a mantra while you walk such as "I am alive and getting stronger every day!" or "I am healthy!" or "I am supercharged now!" or "I am grateful!"

REMEMBER YOUR FAMILY AND FRIENDS ARE NEW TO THIS PROCESS, TOO

When you're feeling overwhelmed with the changes you're making, keep this in mind: it's difficult to be dependent and restricted. It is easy to become frustrated or to lash out, especially at those closest to you. Your family and friends and caregivers are trying to help you and are not sure what or how is the best way to support you. You all will have a settling-in process. Remember that each day will get better, and soon you will be living with new healthy habits that will be lifelong.

> Knowing that you are still here means you have work to do, and your job on this Earth as a human is not done yet.

It's easy to get caught up in fear, worry and doubt. These are valid feelings, but they will not allow you to progress. Your surgery is meant to be a teacher. Channel the worry, doubt and fear to question: What is this experience teaching you? To be patient? To be self-aware? To make your health a priority? To re-think your values? What is this experience teaching your family and friends?

SEEK OUT SUPPORT

Surgery can be traumatic. You could very well have PTSD (Post-Traumatic Stress Disorder), and if you are concerned, please let your doctor know so this can be addressed. It may feel like you are alone and you are scared, and despite the most helpful attempts by friends and family, they have no idea how you feel. Do seek out support groups. Depression is very real for cardiac patients (and their caregivers), and it is important to tackle this emotional and mental hurdle also, as much as your physical wound, in your recovery plan.

IT IS SO IMPORTANT TO MONITOR YOUR THOUGHTS AND FOCUS ON GRATITUDE AND POSITIVITY

Instead of "I had this surgery, I cannot do X, Y and Z," try out new ways of thinking like "Wow—not only did I make it through the surgery, I appreciate every day with new eyes." Allow your tears and emotions to come out. Let them be honored. Grieving is real. If you need help, the act of saying "I need help" can be freeing and ease your mind knowing that your path is not a solo one. You will move back and forth through the stages of grief.

Mentally shift to a perspective of moving forward rather than getting stuck in a bad moment. This life experience will get smaller and smaller in your life's rear view mirror the more you move forward to a healthier future.

DON'T BE AFRAID TO TELL PEOPLE "THANKS FOR YOUR INPUT, I'M GOOD!"

People love to give unsolicited advice, and it is okay to decline it. This is your experience and you can proceed forward in your recovery in a way that works best for you and makes you most comfortable.

> **A word about visitors when you get home from the hospital:**
> Even phone calls and the energy you use in speaking on the phone may zap your energy. It is okay to not talk to someone. This is your time to focus on yourself and your healing. Rest is very important at this time. Don't be afraid to ask for things if you need them. Let people know that if they really want to help you, you would appreciate it if they could: _____. Then, name it. People do want to help, and this will make them feel better while at the same time easing your recovery. Make room for those who bring you energy, not those who drain your energy.

COUGH AND TAKE DEEP BREATHS

Coughing is very important to clear excess mucous out of your lungs and to prevent pneumonia. You will have a splint pillow to hold over your chest to splint and support your chest when you cough. Hopefully you will need your pillow to splint your chest because of laughter. Yes, laughter is good medicine! Feel-good hormones are released when you laugh.

Bonus recognition: If you smoked before, you are now an ex-smoker from your hospital stay. If you are having a hard time with nicotine withdrawal, ask your doctor about using a nicotine patch.

SIT UP IN A CHAIR AS MUCH AS POSSIBLE

Take short walks around the house to start, with assistance. Remember, you will build up your strength gradually each day, so don't push yourself.

WALKING IS EXCELLENT EXERCISE

Start slowly and pace yourself. Start with 5 minutes at a time, a few times a day. In bad weather, you may want to go to a mall in the morning before it gets crowded. Check in at the mall to see if they have any formal organized mall walking groups, or create your own. You will also want to check if the mall has secured COVID-19 protections, (if still applicable) and mindfully physically distance and protect yourself as needed. Do not use a treadmill or exercise equipment until approved by your doctor. Discuss any fitness programs or sports activities with your cardiologist, to get their medical clearance.

As for everyone, if you have shortness of breath or chest pain, palpitations or irregular heartrate, feel dizzy, have unusual or severe chest pain or you feel unwell, stop what you are doing and call your doctor immediately, or if you need to, call 9-1-1. Avoid activities such as shoveling snow, swimming, playing tennis, golf or other aerobic sports until you check with your doctor.

Enjoy building up your walking with a buddy or a family member. Having someone accompany you can put you at ease. Plan your route in advance. Do not wear headphones, earbuds or anything that will distract you from traffic, or from the silent electric bikes that food delivery people and commuters now use. Look both ways, even on a one-way street, as many bicyclists go the wrong way. Be aware and alert to your surroundings. Make sure you are hydrated and also bring water with you on your walks. Do not walk in the highest heat of the day, especially in the summer.

RANGE OF MOTION

Make sure you receive range of motion instructions and any other restrictions from your doctor. It takes about six weeks for the breastbone to heal. You will receive a list of restrictions and ways to mobilize your body. Slowly, you will progress in your range of motion.

DO NOT DRIVE A CAR FOR SIX WEEKS AFTER SURGERY

Get driving clearance from your doctor. You can be a passenger in a car. Enjoy being driven around. You may have a new assignment as a navigator!

FOLLOW YOUR DOCTORS' INSTRUCTIONS FOR POST-OP CARE

Take a shower every day, gently cleaning your incisions with mild soap and warm water. To avoid infection, do not submerge into water. This includes no pools, no baths, no swimming at the beach, no hot tub, and no submersion of your hands and arms in water (you may have had a central line placed in your wrist) until you are cleared by your doctor.

WEIGH YOURSELF EVERY DAY

Record it in the space provided in your daily journal. Weigh yourself without clothing, after waking up and using the bathroom, before you eat or drink in the morning. Keep track of your daily weight in this journal. Tell your doctor if you have a weight gain or loss of greater than 5 pounds in 2–3 days. Ask your doctor what his/her parameters of weight gain are for you to be monitoring.

MONITOR YOUR SURGICAL WOUND(S)

Check for swelling, redness, warmth, tenderness, pus, drainage, separation of the edges of your incision, or if you have chills or fever. Call your doctor if any of these symptoms occur. Steri-strips (tape), clips, staples or stiches will be removed by your doctor. It should take 2–4 weeks for your incision to heal. Do not lift anything heavier than 5 pounds, or as directed, and until cleared by your doctor.

MONITOR BOTH CALVES FOR ANY PAIN AND EXCESS SWELLING

Notify your doctor if you have pain in your calves. Do not rub or massage the area as there could be a clot. Let the doctors assess your leg in person. You may have swelling in a donor site leg. Keep that leg elevated. The swelling should gradually go down. If you are concerned, do not hesitate to contact or go see your doctor.

ASSUME A HEART-HEALTHY NUTRITION PROGRAM

You will be starting this book now if you haven't before surgery, and you will be introduced to a healing program with plant-based nutrition. Adhere to fluid restrictions if you have them. Ask your doctor how much water you can drink each day. If you are diabetic, remain on your diabetic diet for now, until you have read the information for diabetics in this book and as approved by your doctor.

DENTAL CARE AND OTHER MEDICAL PROCEDURES

Alert all doctors and dentists if you have had heart valve surgery or congenital heart defects repaired. You must take special protections to prevent endocarditis, an infection in the heart. You will need to take antibiotics before and after any dental work, surgery or invasive procedure. Ask your doctor when you can resume routine dental care and cleaning. If you develop a fever or sore throat, ask your doctor if you need antibiotics. If you are on a blood thinner, you will need to come in for frequent blood tests and follow up visits with your doctor.

TRAVELING

Do not take any long trips or plan any trips or plane flights without first speaking with your doctor about it. Ensure you have an adequate amount of your medications to take with you on a trip.

PAIN CONTROL

Have pain medications *prior* to getting out of bed, having a dressing change, or using your incentive spirometer if it causes pain. Pain affects your vital signs. Don't wait for your pain to become so great that you are chasing it with medication. Uphold and then gradually lengthen the time frames on the frequency of taking the pain meds. If you are upholding the frequency timeframes and still have pain, called "breakthrough pain," your doctor may prescribe an additional pain medication until your next pain medication is due.

POTTY TALK

You may be given a bowel regimen of medications to facilitate your pooping. Remember we don't want to push or force our bowel movement as this can put additional and unnecessary pressure on the heart. If needed, in addition to your bowel regimen, you could use nature's assistance by having prunes or prune juice and dates if it is approved by your doctor. Chances are, if you haven't pooped, you may not be hungry, however your body needs nutrition to support recovery. Make pooping a top priority. Poop is important!

APPETITE

Your taste may also be off from anesthesia and the bypass machine, if you were on it. Little by little, you should see improvement in your taste and appetite. Try smaller meal portions to begin with, as your digestive system may be slowed down from the anesthesia. Choose foods that are healthy and bring you comfort.

> **ALERT!** Do not have grapefruit or grapefruit juice. It affects how the liver metabolizes your medication, possibly making it more or less effective.

Nature's sports drink is coconut water! Coconut water is full of the electrolytes potassium, and magnesium. I really like the refrigerated brands which come straight from the coconut, to the refrigerated section in the market, to your happy taste buds.

Have a banana a day for potassium, after checking with your doctor to ensure that your potassium levels are OK.

GLUCOSE CONTROL

Immediately post-op you may be treated as a diabetic with finger sticks and insulin administration. The liver sends out glucose to help the body have energy after injury such as it perceives from surgery. Why do we want to keep our blood sugar low? Well, bacteria love sugar, the blood glucose, and what do bacteria cause? Infection. And what do we really not want after a surgery? Infection. So what do we need to get in control? Blood glucose. Who doesn't have food if we control glucose? Bacteria! Eventually the liver will realize everything is fine, you are healing OK, and it will stop sending out glucose.

You may also feel very "foggy" or forgetful after your surgery. You may also have low blood sugar. This fogginess may be because you were under anesthesia for a long period of time, and possibly a bypass machine. Make sure you check in with your nurse and doctor about it.

SEXY TIME

Ask your doctor about resuming sexual activity. An important part of your reactivating your spark and sparkle is communication about each partner's needs, concerns, and feelings. When you do get frisky, do not engage in any position that would cause pressure to be placed on your chest. It is important to resume sexual activity as a part of your life as you would any other part of your life, like breathing and eating. This may be scary at first. Share your concerns with your partner.

Speak to your doctor or therapist about your concerns, and seek out information from your support group, but remember everyone's experiences and timelines are unique to them, and yours will be for you.

RETURNING TO WORK

Returning to work will be dependent on the type of surgery you had, your recovery progress, and the type of work you do. Ask your doctor when you can go back to work and while there, secure a letter from your doctor if your company will need information verifying that you were absent for a hospitalization.

When you are ready to go back to work, go back looking and feeling fierce. Get your hair done, get your nails done, ensure things like money and credit cards are in your wallet. Take any medications you need with you. Pack your crystal up to accompany you. Take home-cooked meals for your lunches and snacks. Take it slow, and schedule time to rest each day in breaks. Use your breath work tools. Ensure you have a sweater to stash away in case the temperature is too cold in the office.

> **PRO TIP**: It is a good idea to wear a medical alert bracelet with emergency contact information, allergies, implants and any other special alerts or needs.

ANTICIPATE QUESTIONS YOUR CO-WORKERS MAY HAVE

Maybe you could even have a huddle with them all to avoid the same questions coming at you from multiple sources. People may be hesitant or not know how to interact with you. They will need your reassurance that you are OK. You cannot control how people will react to you, but you can control your response to them. Anticipate questions and have your responses ready. "How are you feeling?" is met with: "Great! My parts are shinier and newer than yours now!" It will take time to understand how the "new you" will cope in your work environment.

PART-TIME AND WORKING FROM HOME

Check with your employer if you can come back part-time, or even work from home at first. Negotiate if you can come back to partial responsibilities. Ask for help if you need it. Not asking for help when you need it puts an additional stressor on you. If you don't ask, then the answer is automatically a "No!" Inform your employer you will need to be going to doctor's appointments so they can anticipate and plan for your absence.

TAKE YOUR TIME BEFORE RUSHING BACK TO WORK

This may be a wonderful time to assess if this is really the type of work you want to be doing, or if you would like to pivot in your career now.

Many times, we are tied by our ego to what we do. If what we do as an occupation is taken away, some people have a very difficult time with their identity. Consider that your career is not who you are, it is what you do. Many times we value ourselves and others by what they do and not by who they are. Alan Finger, my ISHTA (Integrated Science of Hatha, Tantra and Ayurveda) yoga teacher said: "We are not what we do… if you take that away from someone, and that is how they identify themselves—then who are they if they cannot do that?" I like this philosophy a lot. It releases a self-limiting ego based thought process. It caused me to rethink from identifying myself as a nurse to identifying as a person who does nursing and who now also writes books. Had I stayed in only the nurse "compartment," I may never have stepped out to write this book for you!

"YOUR WORK IS GOING TO FILL A LARGE PART OF YOUR LIFE, AND THE ONLY WAY TO BE TRULY SATISFIED IS TO DO WHAT YOU BELIEVE IS GREAT WORK. AND THE ONLY WAY TO DO GREAT WORK IS TO LOVE WHAT YOU DO. IF YOU HAVEN'T FOUND IT YET, KEEP LOOKING. DON'T SETTLE. AS WITH ALL MATTERS OF THE HEART, YOU'LL KNOW WHEN YOU FIND IT."

—STEVE JOBS, co-founder, Apple

DEPRESSION AFTER HEART SURGERY

I routinely observed depression in my post-op patients. Depression can be a side effect after a cardiac surgery or heart injury/illness. We have hurt (through a controlled surgery) the heart after all, and the heart is one of the main energy centers of the body. One would think that the feeling would be "Yay—I had a lifesaving surgery and now I have another chance at life!" But this is not always the case. Many cardiac patients become depressed. Why would you feel depressed? There are many reasons, many you may not be aware of. You may feel loss of your old life as you accommodate to new adjustments. You may grieve a loss of your work and how you viewed yourself by your work. You may be upset about the scars you have on your body. You may be upset that you feel weak. You may feel dependent due to a loss of autonomy. You may have emotional trauma from all of these events, and as a result, become depressed. Heck, you may not even know why you feel depressed, but it is important to seek assistance. You don't have to suffer, or hurt alone.

> Remember that all of your scars, the visible wounds or the invisible emotional wounds are symbols of a courageous battle you have won, because you are here.

I honored my patient's scars. Patients who have gone through the tremendous emotional and physical pain from surgery are heroes.

> **You will heal. Give yourself time.**

SOME SIGNS OF DEPRESSION:

- Little interest or pleasure in doing things
- Trouble falling asleep or staying asleep
- Feeling down or hopeless
- Feeling tired or having little energy
- Poor appetite or overeating
- Feeling bad about yourself
- Trouble concentrating
- Thoughts of hurting yourself
- Thoughts you would be better off dead
- Fear of another event
- Struggling to get out of bed in the mornings
- Missing or cancelling scheduled commitments

You may be dependent on others for help right now, and that can be difficult, especially for someone who has always been very independent. Keep reminding yourself that you are getting better and stronger every day, and you will move to greater autonomy and independence again.

Your body has endured the trauma akin to a "controlled car accident." Surgically, your body was traumatized. That is a big life event. You also may have suffered mentally from your thoughts in anticipation of the surgery.

Your main energy center of your body has been altered and it needs to heal. If we think about acupuncture, Chinese medicine, energy healing, yoga, reiki, and massage, all of these sciences have honored the energy centers of the body. The heart happens to be the bridge from your upper energy centers, your mind, intuition, thoughts, spirituality, and feelings, to your lower energy centers comprised of your ego, sexuality, safety, and security. When we have a disruption in this energy, this bridge, it can throw things off balance, and the imbalance in your life can lead to depression and anxiety.

Patients have fears of having another cardiac event. This can create tremendous anxiety. Now, though, because you had surgery, you have corrected what was wrong, and actually, you have newer parts than most other people. Avoid being a "Ferris Bueller" (reference from the movie *Ferris Bueller's Day Off*) and getting marked absent, because you *are* here!

Your surgery may even be the demarcation line of "before" your surgery and "after" your surgery that you needed to direct you to living a better and more aware life.

Look in the bathroom mirror at your accountability partner and tell him or her: "I am HERE!"

FIND THE POSITIVE "SILVER LINING" IN YOUR EXPERIENCE

Many of my cardiac surgery patients told me that their surgery or their hospitalization was the catalyst to make them have a better and more fulfilling life, rather than being on "autopilot" every day. What is *your* silver lining? How can you help others to live better by your experience? What changes do you want to make to take your life to a new level? Record your silver lining in your journal.

LET'S TALK ABOUT WHAT A WASTE
OF TIME WORRYING IS

Worry is negative anticipation of something that *may never happen*. Worry drains our time from focusing on healing and on what is going great. We can get into negative downhill spirals when we get mired in negative thoughts. Honor your thoughts when they come up, but do not give them a spot in the parking lot of your mind. Let them drive through! We do not have time for that kind of drama taking up space when we have work to do to heal! What about if you took the time you did in worrying and flipped the thoughts into all the great things that are going to happen for you now? How might your mindset and your energy be impacted by this simple shift in perspective?

> PRO TIP: Move to thoughts of what you are grateful for to replace the thoughts making you anxious or fretful. It takes discipline and practice to control your thoughts. Meditation builds this grateful attitude by helping us control our thoughts.

AVOID HYPOCHONDRIA

Thoughts of still being sick or having a new illness or problem can creep up, but won't serve your goal of living with a positive outlook. Notice if you are monitoring your body to *purposefully seek out* anything going "wrong" from something that is *actually* feeling wrong. Stop and notice how you actually feel. It is easy to get fixated on "What if it happens again?" Well, think of before you got ill, if on a daily basis you were thinking "What if I get sick?" It is not a positive use of your time, and may not ever be an issue. When you do have these thoughts, enable your relaxation response by closing your eyes, breathing in to expand your belly to the count of four, pause and notice the complete inhale, then exhale the belly empty to the count of seven. Repeat seven times. Bring in Prana—your life force energy— to every cell in your body. Notice how you feel after your breath work.

TIME FOR US TO CALL IN SOME POSITIVE AFFIRMATIONS!

"IF YOU TALK TO YOUR BODY, IT WILL LISTEN."
—DR. BERNIE SIEGEL, pediatric surgeon, author

MENTALLY OR OUT LOUD STATE THE FOLLOWING AFFIRMATIONS TO YOURSELF:

- I am: Getting stronger every day
- I am: Thriving, not just surviving
- I am: Healing
- I am: Filled with positive white light, giving me energy
- I am: Nourished by my food
- I am: Uplifted by the emotional support of my family and friends
- I am: Accepting what I cannot control
- I am: Focused on the positives around me
- I am: Replacing worried thoughts with grateful thoughts
- I am: Planning fun things to do in my future

YOUR TURN NOW! LET'S ADD A FEW MORE:

I am:

I am:

I am:

> **Reminder:** Know that by putting the information in your *Heart to Soul Cardiac Wellness* book into action, you are empowering yourself to get better, day by day!

GET INVOLVED WITH SUPPORT GROUPS

There is someone else out there looking to buddy up with someone like you to help you over your life speed bump. Could you also be that person for someone getting ready to go through surgery? One of the best ways to feel better about yourself and your sense of purpose is by helping others.

HONOR YOUR FAITH OR RELIGION

Seek out assistance from your spiritual advisor or your faith-based community.

ASK FOR HELP, BE IT PHYSICAL, MENTAL, EMOTIONAL OR SPIRITUAL

This is the time to put ego aside and allow your humanity to appear. People want to help, but they may not want to offend you by offering. Allow someone to make it easier for you while you are building up your independence. Receiving assistance from others allows someone else to feel good about themselves, too! Look in the mirror and state: "I can receive this!"

TALK TO SOMEONE

Your rehab facility or your doctor may be able to recommend you to a person or therapy group. The American Heart Association will have your local chapter information for assistance in finding support.

TRY JOURNALING YOUR THOUGHTS, EXPERIENCES, AND FEELINGS

Sometimes journaling helps to get your feelings out, if you are hesitant to tell someone. You can take this journal to a therapist if you decide to see one. Your thoughts do become your feelings, and this is why it is important to keep positive thoughts. Remember "The Law of Attraction."

DECIDE HOW YOU WANT TO PRESENT YOURSELF

Will you be conducting yourself to be a Cardiac Thriver, or only a survivor? Your body and scars may heal, and you may find your biggest challenge will be your mental thoughts and the actions you take toward recovery and wellness. You have a message you can share with people through your story. You can be an inspiration for others. You are in a position now to regroup and take a new path to health. In addition to lifestyle changes, *accepting* this life event is key to moving forward.

There will always be a "before" and an "after" your cardiac event. Accepting this and coming to terms with it is your new reality. It will affect how you think. The head and the heart and the gut are connected. What you experienced is scary, and can be traumatic. You had a powerful thing happen to you—honor that. You are alive, and you have tools here to help you to be the best version of yourself. Controlling your thoughts is going to take some effort in self-awareness so you can catch yourself when you get into a negative thought spiral. It is a time now to understand how you react to people. Have you been a Type A personality in control of people and situations? Have you had a quick temper? Have you *reacted* instead of *responded*? Take mental inventory and press pause before you make a hasty response; come to your interactions with compassion before you reply, so you don't have a reaction. This is especially true in how you interact with those caring for you.

DON'T BARK AT THOSE TRYING TO HELP YOU; INSTEAD, THANK THEM

They are scared, too, trying to adjust to this new situation, and they probably don't have much direction or support. (Please refer them to the next chapter, dedicated to caregivers.) This is new for them, too. They may have their own trauma. Remember, they were waiting long hours during the operation not knowing what would happen. They were at your bedside when you were on life support or sedated from a surgery. They were cheerleading for you. They may have been praying for you. They went through a very scary time, too. They are coping with their own trauma, and your care and considerations, while still maintaining their own life, work, families and personal commitments. Saying "Thank You" or "I Appreciate You" will really go a long way to anyone who helps you. Take a look at this situation through their eyes for a moment to get their perspective. Everyone is recovering from the same incident, with a different viewpoint. Call forth your compassion for them.

YOU WILL ATTRACT THE RIGHT EMOTIONAL SUPPORT WITH A POSITIVE MINDSET, TOO

Is there a talisman such as a crystal or favorite rock, a medallion or touchstone that you can put out on your work area or carry in your pocket so that you have a reminder to keep you in a positive state? It is really important to find support, whether it be in a friend who also had such an event, or through a support group. We are not just healing your body; we are healing your mental and emotional trauma, too. Keeping a positive outlook will attract even more positivity in the things that come your way. Your talisman can serve as your physical reminder that you are ok.

TAKE IT EASY AND TAKE IT ONE DAY AT A TIME

You can absolutely enjoy every day and thrive. Each day will get better and easier as you heal. Remember that you had a problem, it has been corrected, and you now have this plan for optimization and recovery.

MAKE A LIST OF YOUR QUESTIONS

Have a list of questions you have been compiling for your doctor so you don't forget anything when you are there. Don't forget to bring a note taker with you to record information for you so you can fully absorb what the doctor is telling you. You will be going to follow-up doctor's visits, where you can monitor and celebrate your progress. Your doctor wants to hear about your successes and be a part of your recovery team. Celebrate how far you have come after each check-up.

PLAN AHEAD

Imagine something you are going to enjoy when you get better, and how you will FEEL when you are doing it! Put this activity in your calendar so it is real and it has a date. Consider when you feel up to it:

- Start a walking group. Check to see if your local mall or town has a walking group.

- Resource and attend local open-heart support groups.

- Start your own support group, or see if your doctor's office wants to establish a support program.

- Offer to be a buddy to visit someone who had the same surgery as you for a pre-op or post-op visit in the hospital, or a phone check-in.

What to Expect

IF YOU ARE A PARTNER/ SPOUSE/CAREGIVER

How are you doing as a caregiver? How are you feeling? Caregivers are often overlooked because you are not the focus, your loved one is. You may have your own fears and worries and challenges. You may feel guilt, and you may feel emotionally distraught. I hope the information in the two preceding chapters and what I am sharing here in this chapter can help you as you navigate this new territory. It is vital that you embrace what works best for you. It is easy to isolate yourself and very important that you do seek support offered, so you can share your burden.

As a caregiver, you need your own self-care, too, to ensure you stay healthy and rested so you can be fully present for your loved one. Take care of yourself and remember that you can't be a 24/7 support. You need to rest and take much-needed breaks, too. When visitors come, that is your reminder to take a break. Having a schedule of "Wing Persons" at bedside can offset your presence, allowing you to take time for yourself.

FIRST: CHECK-IN WITH YOUR OWN SELF-CARE

Are you taking care of yourself and your own needs first? A morning meditation and brief walk might be what you need before you roll up your sleeves and dig in so you can be the rock each day for your special person. You cannot give of yourself or be of service to your loved one if you have no energy, just as you cannot drive a car if there is no gas in the tank. *Self-care is your gas.* You also want to make sure that you are eating well and getting adequate rest.

Know that each day will get a little easier as your loved one heals.

Know they will be cranky and that they may even be downright mean. They aren't feeling or looking their best. They may be having trouble coping with their life adjustments. They may be frustrated with their temporary loss of independence, possibly suffering from depression and post-ICU syndromes, post-anesthesia mental fogginess, and even emotional trauma, or PTSD.

Your loved one will be going through a range of emotions from fear, anticipatory fear of another event, worry, shock, guilt, shame, anger, frustration, confusion, and depression. Come to them with compassion and cut them some slack. Do not react immediately if they say something that is hurtful or what you feel is unwarranted. Do not take things personally. They aren't feeling themselves. Try responding with "I hear what you are saying. You are...," reframing or reiterating what they said to make them feel that they are being heard. You can even say "I hear you." and "I am here for you." "You are supported." "Let's work on this together." It is really helpful to bring all this out in the open—the feelings, expressing them, and that you are there as friend, not foe.

Encourage "supportive autonomy," marking each progressive step forward with your recovering heart patient. Celebrate little wins, even if only a "Yay—you got two more steps in today—it's progress!"

Accept only those visitors who will *bring* supportive energy, not *sap* it from your loved one or you.

PREPARE VISITORS

Visitors may be sidelined by what they see versus what they expected to see. It is scary going into a critical care unit, and it might help to prepare them. A few good ground rules to have are "Only good news to be shared." and "Advice on request, not unsolicited." and "No in-depth details on the reason for the hospital stay." I advised visitors to lightly state to the effect that "You got sick, you are in the hospital and you are now getting better!" I once had a patient whose brother came in and blurted out in a thick Brooklyn accent: "Dude! Yo! You freaking passed out cold at the ball game and fell after you paid for your beer and it was crazy and someone did CPR and then the ambulance came and said you had a cardiac arrest." My patient's eyes were opening wider and wider and he was petrified at that point, and needless to say I had to spend the better part of the afternoon calming the patient and offering him emotional support. It's important to keep things light, supportive, and focused on the future.

As a caregiver, be present bedside when the doctors talk to the patient. Know what time (if they have a usual timeframe when they round) the doctors will be there during bedside rounds, so you can hear their report and be able to ask questions so you can be an informed participant in the recovery plan. You are an important member of the recovery team, after all!

CPR:
WHAT THESE THREE
LIFE-SAVING LETTERS MEAN

Everyone should know how to try to save the life of someone who has collapsed, appears lifeless, and is not moving or breathing. Precious moments are lost that could affect their brain and heart if there is inaction or a lack of proper response to help this person. This chapter denotes an explanation of adult CPR. An adult who goes into sudden cardiac arrest (when the heart stops beating entirely or is beating in an uncoordinated, inefficient pattern) has only a short time before their brain cells start to die—possibly resulting in a permanent, irreversible process of brain injury. For the purposes of this guide, we will focus on adult hands-only CPR.

This brief explanation of CPR does not substitute for the content, personal instruction, and certification you would get in a formal CPR class. I encourage you to take a formal class and get certified in CPR.

ACT FAST, BUT BE SAFE

So, what can you do to help this collapsed person? First, consider your own safety. You cannot help others if you are not safe yourself. Take a few seconds to check your location and make sure you are safe—no fuel leaking from a car crash that might erupt into flames, no possibility of carbon monoxide poisoning that caused the person to become unconscious, no sparking loose electrical wires or other obvious safety hazards.

Now, you have come across this seemingly unconscious person, you have assessed the area and determined it is safe to proceed. How do you know this person is really unconscious and clinically dead (no pulse, no breathing) and requires CPR, versus just sleeping off some excess alcohol or drugs? You must check to be sure the person is indeed unresponsive before you start CPR. How? Look at them: are they moving? Do they appear lifeless? Are they lying there gasping? Gasps could be what are called "agonal breaths," which are not adequate respirations, and require CPR intervention.

TAP AND SHOUT

Approach them from behind their head (the safest mode of approach if you are helping a person outdoors in an open area such as on the street), tap both shoulders and shout "Are you OK?" "Are you OK?" and step back. Tap on both shoulders in case the person suffered a stroke or is paralyzed or has no feeling in one of the shoulders. If the person is just sleeping soundly, they will wake up and may become aggressive. Therefore, you are safer if you have approached them from the top of their head and then backed off. If they still appear unresponsive, repeat the tapping and shouting one more time.

CALL 911

Next, call 9-1-1 immediately—get the professionals on the way to help you. If you have someone with you, tell them to call 9-1-1 while you begin CPR. Give the 9-1-1 operator specifics on your location and what the situation is. Tell the operator you are starting CPR and ask for them to send paramedics. If there are other people present to assist, designate a specific person to get an Automated External Defibrillator (AED). Usually the nearest restaurant will have one. How to use the AED will be explained later in this chapter.

By performing CPR, you are maintaining the heart's circulatory capacities at some of its normal output—enough to perfuse vital organs to sustain life until the AED arrives and can be used. Don't waste time: you need to start CPR immediately. Limit interruptions for optimal blood flow, otherwise the momentum you have built up with your compressions will be significantly diminished.

LAY PERSON FLAT ON BACK

In order to start CPR, the unconscious person must be flat on their back on a hard, firm surface. You cannot do CPR on a person in bed—the mattress below them will absorb your compressions and CPR will not be effective. You may need to roll the person to get them into the proper position. Always protect their head and neck while you get them into position, as they may have fallen and have an injury you cannot see. If others are present, get them to help you position the person properly.

HANDS-ON ONLY CPR

You only need to perform chest compressions—hands-on only CPR. Effective compressions can offer some oxygen into the lungs during the proper chest recoil after each compression. Be sure to let the chest rise completely between compressions for lung expansion.

PROPER POSITION IS KEY

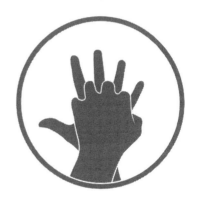

Kneel alongside the person, placing your knees right next to their body, rapidly rip open their outer garments, open their shirt, if applicable move their bra out of the way, and place the heel of your hand in the middle of their chest on the sternum (breast bone) in an imaginary line where their armpits will come together in the middle of the chest. For most adults, that spot corresponds to the mid-nipple line. If your victim is an elderly or obese woman with sagging breasts, you must rely on the armpit measurement, otherwise you will be too low on the chest. You need to rest the heel of your hand on the upper half of the sternum. If you place your hand too low on the sternum, you run the risk of pressing down on a small bone called the "xiphoid process" that lies near the lower half of the sternum and which, when pressed, may cut into the liver below and cause internal bleeding.

PUSH HARD, PUSH FAST

Once you are in place, interlock your hands, lock your elbows, and keep your arms straight. Immediately begin compressions at the rate of at least 100 per minute. Your compressions should be about 2 inches deep. You can practice how deep and hard to push by pressing down on a bathroom scale to generate 80 pounds of pressure. Push hard and push fast. Maintain a solid rhythm. The rhythm should be fast, akin to the beat of the famous (and appropriate) song by the Bee Gees titled "Stayin' Alive". Allow for full chest recoil so the blood you are manually moving can circulate throughout the body, and the lungs can take in air. If possible, have someone else who knows CPR switch with you after 2 minutes so you can have a break. Performing CPR is tiring work and you will need the break in order to have the strength to give adequate compressions.

GET THE AED

Where can an AED be found? AEDs are usually located where large numbers of people are present such as airports, bus and train stations, movie theatres, gyms, restaurants, sports arenas, office buildings and schools. As an exercise for yourself, mindfully observe if the places you frequent have AEDs. They are usually mounted on the wall in a box, and an alarm will sound once you open the box. The defibrillator is a machine that will shock the heart, hopefully back into an organized, functional rhythm, via the pads you place on the chest and the electrical shock, if designated.

HOW THE AED WORKS

If the AED arrives before the emergency medical personnel, turn on the machine, or just open up the apparatus and observe if there is a power button or it turns on automatically. The AED will "talk to you," and walk you through all the steps in its operation. You will place the two pads on the victim's bare chest following the placement directions drawn on each pad. The victim's chest should be dry and ideally hairless. On a very hairy person, if there is a second set of pads available, open and use them to pull the chest hair off quickly, by applying then ripping off the pads. Then, apply the other new set of pads. Ensure the pads you apply are appropriate; adult pads for an adult and pediatric pads for a child. Follow the pictures on the pads. Plug in the connector and follow the voice prompts. Do not stop CPR; work the pads around the process. Only stop CPR when directed to do so by the AED; that is when the AED is analyzing the heart rhythm. If advised by the AED to stop CPR and to "shock" the person, yell "Clear!" and look carefully at the person and others at the scene to make sure no one is touching the person—that all is clear before you press the blinking "shock" button. Otherwise, others may be shocked as well as the intended person—a very dangerous situation that can stop the heart of the other person touching the victim.

TURNING OVER CARE

Once the EMTs and paramedics arrive, turn the care over to them, but be sure you stay to offer additional help if necessary. Be proud that you have been a key player in the chain of survival that has hopefully saved a life.

We encourage you or a family member to get formally trained in CPR. You can go to CPR.HEART.ORG or the American Heart Association website to sign up for a CPR class.

ORGAN DONATION

Organ donation is a difficult subject to talk about. No one wants to talk about dying, but the fact is that we all do one day. If our death happened due to an unexpected situation, wouldn't it be amazing to have a part of you be able to continue living on to help another person?

I have cared for patients who were donors, and while their body in its appearance still looked viable, their brain function was gone, meaning they were clinically unable to support their life functions. I remember one patient I was maintaining on life support because he was an organ donor. The many different teams that were needed to harvest certain organs had to be well coordinated, and his organs were successfully transplanted. Another patient had arranged for a direct liver donation transplant in advance, as he was a match—think of this type of "planning ahead" when you know your friend is in need and you planned for him in the event you had an unexpected end to your life.

Our unit got letters of thanks from families and organizations for helping in the care of these donor patients and in the emotional support given to their families. A death is never easy, but knowing someone was going to help other people was the silver lining we looked to.

One of my favorite floats in the Rose Parade on New Year's Day in Pasadena, California, is the Organ Donor float. Riding on the float are organ donor recipients standing in front of a picture of the person they received life from. That float always makes my eyes mist up.

Gary (who wrote the foreword to this book) is on the wait list for a heart transplant at the time of this writing. Dr. Lima, who wrote the back cover endorsement for this book, is the Heart Transplant Surgeon on Gary's incredible Heart Transplant Team.

Your organ donation could save another person's life. You can register to be an organ donor with the Department of Motor Vehicles when you update your driver's license or on www.RegisterMe.org.

"WE MAKE A LIVING BY WHAT WE GET, BUT WE MAKE A LIFE BY WHAT WE GIVE."

—SIR WINSTON CHURCHILL, former Prime Minister of the United Kingdom

---

More than ever, we all need to take care of and support each other. Taking the time to learn CPR could mean you can save another's life. I had many patients who are still thriving today, because someone they didn't even know stepped up to give them CPR, before trained medical professionals arrived on the scene.

It was always so rewarding to my patient and their families when first responders circled back to the hospital a day or two after a patient had fallen ill to see how the person they had resuscitated was doing. It brought tears to all our eyes to witness that caring and human connection, and that very feeling is what inspired me to become a nurse. It was by serendipity that I was selected to be a cardiac ICU nurse. It could have been any ICU, but it was very special—the CCU.

AFTERWORD

BY SOHAH N. IQBAL, MD

Interventional Cardiologist

Mass General Brigham Salem Hospital/Mass General Hospital

Knowledge is power, action is power, and this book, Mary Yuter's *Heart to Soul Cardiac Wellness* gives individuals both the knowledge and actionable items to create meaningful change, hence giving us power over our own cardiac health. As a cardiologist who puts stents in blocked arteries and prescribes medicines, I try to take the extra few minutes to discuss lifestyle changes. My patients always want more time and have more questions and I know a few minutes is not enough to educate and empower them. I truly believe there is more we in health care can do to help our patients take care of themselves. And in my mind, this is that something more!

As individuals who inevitably become patients, most of us fall into two buckets—those of us who believe heart disease can't happen to us and the other that believes there is nothing we can do to prevent it. Whichever side of the spectrum you are on, this book is a resource that gives you tools on how to decrease your risk and possibly alter the course of your disease processes. There is a lot of literature out there on this subject, but Mary's book brings dispersed information together in one place in an easy to read and manageable way.

In this book you are literally getting part of Mary's Heart and Soul. This is her passion project, with many years of hard work and dedication behind this piece of work. Mary has always invested herself in every patient. She went beyond their critical care needs and acknowledged their physical and emotional well-being. Wellness is a part of who Mary is and she wanted to expand her reach from her individual patients to all of you. She knocked on doors of leaders, she attended conference after conference to network and discuss her ideas with experts around the world. She put in the time while working full time as a CCU (Cardiac Care Unit) nurse in a very busy city hospital cardiac center to get the training, understand the evidence, and study the data around lifestyle change and its lasting effects.

Mary did the work to help you. Now that you have had a chance to read this book once, put in the time to translate it into practice. Decide what are things you think are doable and focus on them to start. Mary gives you permission to take this step by step for a reason. Don't take this wealth of information for granted. I am firm believer of change in daily practice leading to habit. I personally started with eating vegetarian lunches and taking the stairs instead of taking theelevator at work and now it is fully ingrained in my day today routine. It takes work in the beginning and Mary acknowledges that. What a useful, engaging, and powerful guide! This is a true resource—as if Mary was right there with you on your journey.

ACKNOWLEDGMENTS

Mary: I am so grateful for the support necessary to create *Heart to Soul Cardiac Wellness*. This book would not have been here in your hands, were it not for Dr. Sohah Iqbal, who believed in me and encouraged me to keep going. Thank you to Bernice for coming to our fireside chats with a smile, even after your long days. Special big love and gratitude to Remi, for your support from day one of *Heart to Soul Cardiac Wellness*, your feisty spirit, your loving eye rolls of "patience" while taking out my extra spaces and for being such a sparkle in my life, making me so very proud of you every day. To my "doctor" Chimpy, thank you for your keen eye and advice, for your cheerleading and for taking such beautiful care of me while this book was created. I am so grateful to you. Tremendous gratitude to my Muse and heroine Reeb, and her rock Miguel, because you overcame and you are such an example of "Living your best life." "Terra Firma" to the fabulous Banan for regularly checking in on me from your car, your sofa, or your lounge chair in Palm Springs, with your delightful phone calls and adorable laugh. Thank you so much to my inspirational friend, Gary Sherman, DMD, who shows up to life daily with a twinkle in his eye and a smile on his face. You all have been by my side every step of the way, believing in my vision, cheering, listening, supporting, smiling and helping me. Thank you to all of my friends who are also my family. You all make *my* heart beat happily!

Ed Mylett, a very special thank you for being such a light for me to look up to during the making of this book, and for your incredibly inspiring posts which every day seemed to be speaking straight to me. Warm gratitude to my own doctors, Dr. Lutsky and Dr. Dunham for partnering with me for my health and wellness. Shout out to vegan champion and plant-based cook Stephanie De Marco, all the way from Louisiana, for her savvy plant-based input. Thank you to my wonderful SCORE mentor, Jill Friedlander, who was my oyster, dispensing pearls of publishing wisdom to me. Thank you to Domini Dragoone for her creative vision in launching this book into formal design copy. Namaste and thank you to my yogi friend and my "Cover Girl" photographer Laura Jane Brett, who made it so easy to fall into your lens.

I must also acknowledge my former colleagues with whom I spent over thirteen years of my life; my Nurse sisters and brothers, Doctors, PAs, NPs, the fearless Respiratory Therapists, Pharmacists, all the CCU, ICU, Cath Lab, CVPACU staff, the PCAs and PCTs, Phlebotomy, Housekeepers, Foodservice, Clerks, Administrators, Union Reps, and all the many other ancillary hospital staff who taught me so much and who work so very hard each day, kindly caring for the sickest of the sick in NYC.

Bernice: Heartfelt thanks to all my steadfast friends—you know who you are—who helped me along to way with sound advice, inspiration, encouragement and generosity of spirit.

ABOUT THE AUTHORS

Mary Yuter lives in New York City, and her natural habitat is on the beach, engrossed in a wellness book or swimming in the ocean. Mary, a mermaid at heart, collects sea glass and shells. Mary loves yoga, exploring health food stores and crystal shops, cooking, biking, skiing and taking long road trips with great music, lots of snacks, and chewy conversation. Mary is currently checking-off two items on her bucket list: learning to play drums, and making sea glass necklaces. Mary is passionate about helping people improve their wellness holistically, while honoring the science of Western medicine. Mary is inspired by the determination of the human spirit and in people's life stories.

Bernice Pass-Stern, author of the CPR content, is a health educator with an extensive history as a CPR instructor-trainer and regional faculty member with the American Heart Association. Bernice is a native New Yorker who has embraced community service as a means for educating others about health promotion, wellness and disease prevention. As a Captain in the New York City Auxiliary Police Program, she has taught CPR and first aid to thousands of other New York volunteers over the last 35 years. Bernice loves working with aspiring nursing students, running marathons, hiking in the mountains, caring for animals, collecting art and does fashion modeling as an advocate to fight ageism and stereotyping.

RESOURCE BOUTIQUE

"KNOWLEDGE ISN'T POWER UNTIL IT IS APPLIED."
—DALE CARNEGIE, writer, lecturer

Please enjoy this curated selection of wellness resources, from healthy nutrition sites, meditations, healing and healthy lifestyle aids, books, websites, podcasts, movies, and empowering holistic tools to help you optimize your vibrant life energy.

> **Bonus Gifts!** As a *Heart to Soul Cardiac Wellness* reader, receive the gift of a discount on your purchase using discount code HEART where noted, for healing and wellness products I recommend on my website www.hearttosoulcw.com under the heading "Wellness Boutique."

Supportive, Informational, and Inspirational Websites

hearttosoulcw.com

pcrm.org

drmiltonmillsplantbasednation.com

downstate.edu/plant-based

cardiosmart.org

childrenshealthdefense.org

brownvegan.com

blackvegansrock.com

heartrhythmalliance.org

ppmny.org

abcardio.org

badassvegan.com

health.harvard.edu

diabetes.org

fatmanrants.com

Drheart2heart.net

wickedhealthyfood.com

drnorthrup.com

ewg.org

peta.org

drfuhrman.com

sciencedaily.com

mindbodygreen.com

wholegrainscouncil.org

ted.com

nutritionfacts.org

mendedhearts.org

heartmath.com

heart.org

veganuary.com

vegansociety.com

plantbasednews.org

milliondollarvegan.com

womenheart.org

clevelandclinic.org

knowdiabetesbyheart.org

forksoverknives.com

howtogettheguy.com

bylr.co

edmylett.com

richroll.com

masteringdiabetes.org

blackvegfest.com

honeybeeherbs.com

jesseitzler.com

orgoneenergyfields.com

thecoppervessel.com

dinaberrin.com

Vegan Food Recipe and Meal Planning Websites

pcrm.org

plantpoweredkitchen.com

vegansociety.com

EatRight.org

thehungrychickpea.com

straightupfood.com

cookingwithplants.com

goodcatchfoods.com

thissavoryvegan.com

Apps You Can Use to Verify if a Home or Body Product Is Healthy

(You can also check your beauty and makeup products here!)

Think Dirty Think Dirty-Shop Clean

EWG Healthy Living Environmental Working Group

Recommendations from My Bookshelf

Please note: The authors listed below have written many other books than those listed here, so please look for their other books, too!

UnDo It! by Dr. Dean Ornish and Anne Ornish

Healthy at Last: A Plant-Based Approach to Preventing and Reversing Diabetes and Other Chronic Illnesses by Eric Adams

Saving Women's Hearts by Martha Gulati, MD

Protein Aholic: How Our Obsession with Meat is Killing Us and What We Can Do About it by Garth Davis, MD

Heart to Beat by Brian Lima, MD

The Trifecta of Health by Angie Sadeghi, MD and Dan Holtz, with Matt Bennett

The Blue Zones: Nine lessons for living longer by Dan Buettner

Reverse Heart Disease Now by Stephen Sinatra, MD

Mastering Diabetes by Cyrus Khambatt and Robby Barbaro

How Not to Die by Michael Greger, MD

Identically Different by Tim Spector

The Pleasure Trap by Doug Lisle, MD

The Cheese Trap by Neil Barnard, MD

The Alzheimer's Solution by Ayesha Sherzai, MD and Dean Sherzai, MD

Prevent and Reverse Heart Disease by Caldwell Esselstyn, MD

Too Young for a Heart Attack by Stu Segal

Heart Smart for Women by Jennifer H. Mieres, MD, FACC and Stacey Rosen, MD, FACC

Heart Attack Proof by Michael Ozner, MD

The Whole Heart Solution by Joel Kahn, MD

The Heart Healers by James Forrester, MD

Cleanse to Heal by Anthony William

Coping with Heart Surgery and Bypassing Depression by Carol Cohan, MA, June B. Pimm, PhD, James R. Jude, MD

Back to Life After a Heart Crisis by Mark Wallack, MD and Jamie Colby

The Patient's Guide to Heart Valve Surgery by Adam Pick

The China Study by T. Colin Campbell, PhD and Thomas M. Campbell, MD

Books for Mental Health, Inspiration, and Personal Growth

Any of the motivational books by Dr. Wayne Dyer

A Mind of Your Own by Dr. Kelly Brogan

Breaking the Habit of Being Yourself by Dr. Joe Dispenza

Living With The Monks by Jesse Itzler

#Maxout Your Life by Ed Mylett

The Tapping Solution by Nick Ortner

Healthy, Happy, Sexy: Ayurveda Wisdom for Modern Women by Katie Silcox

Absolute Beauty by Dr. Pratima Raichur

The Silver Disobedience Playbook by Dian Griesel

Women's Bodies, Women's Wisdom by Dr. Christiane Northrup

The Four Agreements: A Practical Guide to Personal Freedom by Don Miguel Ruiz

The Alchemist: A Fable About Following Your Dream by Paulo Coelho

Emotional Agility: Get Unstuck, Embrace Change and Thrive in Work and Life by Susan David

The Genius Life: Heal Your Mind, Strengthen Your Body, and Become Extraordinary by Max Lugavere

Think Like A Monk: Train Your Mind for Peace and Purpose Every Day by Jay Shetty

The Art of Healthy Living: How Good Nutrition and Improved Well-being Leads to Increased Productivity, Vitality and Happiness by Denise Kelly

I USED TO BE A MISERABLE F*CK: An Everyman's Guide to a Meaningful Life by John Kim

How to do the Work: Recognize Your Patterns, Heal from Your Past + Create Your Self by Dr. Nicole LePera

Books about Crystals and Essential Oils

Crystal Healer by Phillip Permutt

Crystal Energy: 150 Ways to Bring Success, Love, Health and Harmony into Your Life by Mary Lambert

Crystal Muse by Heather Askinose and Timmi Jandro

Just the Essentials by Adina Gilgore

National Geographic Complete Guide to Herbs and Spices by Kelley Edkins

Journaling

Nothing fancy required; simple wire bound pads or notebooks from the store will do. You can individualize a simple spiral bound book with stickers and your own doodles if you want. Stationery and bookstores online have beautiful ones; some are even leather bound.

The Cosmic Journal by Yanik Silver
Skinny Bitchin' by Rory Friedman and Kim Barnouin

Books to Help You on Your Healing Path with Food

The Vegan Starter Kit by Neal Barnard, MD
The Vegucation of Robin: How Real Food Saved My Life by Robin Quivers
Meat is for Pussies: A How-to Guide for Dudes Who Want to Get Fit, Kick Ass, and Take Names by John Joseph
Mad Cowboy by Howard F. Lyman
Eat for Life by Joel Fuhrman, MD
How to Go Vegan by Veganuary
The Plant Based Solution by Joel Kahn, MD
The Pantry Principle: How to Read the Label and Understand What's Really in Your Food by Mira Dessy
Formerly Known as Food: How the Industrial Food System Is Changing Our Minds, Bodies, and Culture by Kristin Lawless
Fast Food Nation by Eric Schlosser
By Any Greens Necessary: A Revolutionary Guide for Black Women Who Want to Eat Great, Get Healthy, Lose Weight and Look Phat by Tracye McQuirter, MPH
Sistah Vegan by A. Breeze Harper, PhD
Crazy Sexy Diet, Eat Your Veggies, Ignite your spark, and Live Like You Mean It! by Kris Carr
Becoming Vegan by B. Davis, RD
Dirty Vegan: Another Bite by Matt Pritchard
The Everything Vegan Pregnancy Book by Reed Mangels, PhD, RD

Vegan Cookbooks

The Wicked Healthy Cookbook by Chad Sarno, Derek Sarno, and David Joachim

Afro-Vegan: Farm Fresh African, Caribbean & Southern Flavors, Remixed by Bryant Terry

Ageless Vegan by Tracye McQuirter, MPH with Mary McQuirter

Eat to Live Cookbook by Joel Fuhrman, MD

Street Vegan by Adam Sobel

The No Meat Athlete by Matt Frazier and Stepfanie Romine

How Not to Die Cookbook by Michael Greger, MD

Wait. That's Vegan?! by Lisa Dawn Angerame

How to be Vegan and Keep Your Friends by Annie Nichols

The Oh She Glows Cookbook by Angela Liddon

The Yoga Kitchen by Kimberly Parsons

The Plantpower Way by Rich Roll and Julie Piatt

Forks Over Knives the Cookbook by Del Sroufe

Crazy Sexy Diet by Kriss Carr

Quick and Easy Vegan Comfort Foods by Alicia Simpson

Sweet Potato Soul by Jenne Claiborne

Ayurvedic Cooking for Self Healing by Usha Lad and Dr. Vasant Lad

Inspirational and Informative Podcasts

(Check out their online and Instagram sites, too!)

Ed Mylett

Brain Health and Beyond

The Doctor's Farmacy

Nutrition Rounds

The Angry Therapist

Broken Brain

Rich Roll

The Plant Proof Podcast

The Heart of the Matter

Bulletproof Radio

Feel Better Live More

Kwik Brain

The Medical Medium

Glass Half Healthy

Single on Purpose

OG Talk

Meditation Channels Online

Boho Beautiful

The Copper Vessel

Simplehappyzen

Goodful

Yogini Melbourne

The Mindful Movement

Jason Stephens

Unlock Your Life

Monterey Bay Aquarium Medit-Ocean

Purely Lucy

Bob Baker

Rising Higher Meditation

Live the Life You Love

Meditation Apps

Calm

Breathe

Headspace

Insight Timer (free)

The Breathing App (free)

More Movies I Highly Recommend

They're Trying to Kill Us

Fast Food Nation

Eating You Alive

Vegucated

Simply Raw

Code Blue

Dominion

Rotten

Stink!

Made in the USA
Middletown, DE
20 November 2022

15420213R00212